Dear Jane

Train hard!.
Lots of love

[signature]

AUGUST 2009

Martin Day has other books and DVD'S available at:

www.MartinDayFitness.com

BOOKS:

Secrets of Fighting Fit Exposed: Battle-Proven Conditioning Exercises for Strength Flexibility and Fitness

Defend Yourself! Ketsugo: Complete Self – Defence

DVDS:

Fighting Fit: Upper Body (chest and arms) Workout

Fighting Fit: Mid-Section (abs and back) Workout

Fighting Fit: Lower Body (legs and core strength) Workout

Uncensored Elite Unarmed Combat: Grabs and Pressure Points

Uncensored Elite Unarmed Combat: Holds and Strikes

Uncensored Elite Unarmed Combat: Weapons

Killer Power Kicks and Punches: Winning Martial Arts Techniques

Ultimate Fighting Fit Flexibility Techniques

Basic Katas (Forms)

Advanced Black Belt Katas (Forms)

 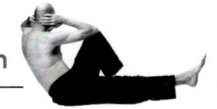

FIGHTING FIT ABS

Battle Proven Exercises That Build Steel Hard, Powerful and Impact Proof Abs

A Martin Day Book / Original Copyright © MMVII

All Rights reserved

First Edition July 2009

ISBN: 978-0-9803845-3-6

PRINTED IN AUSTRALIA

Martin Day Publications

Suite 8, Noosa Boardroom
28 Eenie Creek Rd
Noosaville
Queensland 4566
Australia

E-mail: info@MartinDayFitness.com
Phone: +61 (7) 5430 6662
Fax: + 61 (7) 5430 6677

Disclaimer

Please note that the advice and exercises featured in this book may be very exhaustive and difficult for some of you. If this is the case then you, the reader should consult a physician prior to following these exercises.

The author, creators, producers, participants, advertisers and distributors of this instructional book is not responsible or liable in any manner whatsoever for any injury or loss in connection with the exercises and nutritional advice contained herein.

 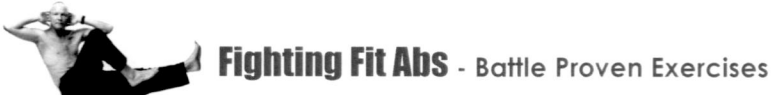

Acknowledgements

Books don't get finished without the help and assistance of many people.

This book is dedicated to my Dad who sadly died whilst I was writing this book. I thank him for being so very strong both in body and in mind, never giving up and for giving me the inspiration to achieve many great things in my life and for being my role model.

We all miss you very much Dad.

Many thanks to Phill Jackson Photography   **www.NoosaPhotographer.com**
for having the expertise and patience to get me to be more photogenic!

To Carol Déjean-Manvill **www.siennarosedesigns.com.au** and John Banitsiotis **www.mediamojo. com.au** for putting the book together for me....

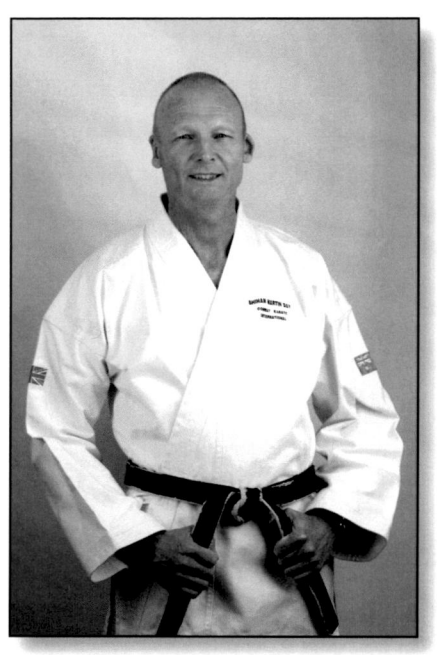

ABOUT THE AUTHOR:

Martin Day was born in Sussex, England in 1955 and moved to Australia in 2004. He says he is "not a hero" but he has been awarded active service and campaign medals gained through his military career with elite British Army combat units for twenty years. Some of the units he has trained include Special Forces, the Coldstream Guards, the Ghurkha's, The Parachute Regiment and Royal Marines.

A lot of his time was also spent abroad training Australian, New Zealand, American and Canadian armed forces. Martin has always been interested in health, physical fitness and anything associated with core conditioning and cardiovascular fitness. His other passion is learning and teaching self defense and martial arts; especially freestyle sport karate. He has excelled in martial arts and various sports and he is the holder of many International titles. He has a reputation as a no nonsense sportsman and he has dominated everything that he has wanted to achieve and continues to be extremely focused on being the best he can be and to also help others to be the best.

During his military career he fought for the Army as a member of the Army boxing team and he is a qualified boxing coach. He has also had significant success in cross country running, 1500 and 5000 metres, swimming and Olympic distance triathlon. His many other qualifications include personal trainer, ASA swimming teacher, track and field coach, physical training, unarmed combat, pressure points and arrest and restraint techniques Instructor. He has taught survival, military tactics, weapons and other military and civilian subjects throughout the world.

In 1975 he was identified as the "youngest patrol commander in the British Army" and went on to gain high rank and service recognition before he left his Army career behind in October 1993. After studying for a physical education degree at Chichester University in West Sussex he set up a covert surveillance and close protection organisation. In 1996 he designed and implemented his own dynamic self defence and martial arts system for adults and children of all abilities. His training system is now practiced worldwide and it reflects his impressive physical ability and dynamic no nonsense lead from the front approach. He has taught his skills to the Police, youth groups and martial arts organisations in various parts of the World and remains in great demand.

Martin Day has been awarded the title of Shihan (Master Instructor of his own training system) and currently holds the rank of 5th Dan Karate Black Belt. He has been featured many times in Combat, Black Belt, Traditional Karate, Martial Arts Illustrated and Blitz magazines worldwide and has been interviewed on radio.

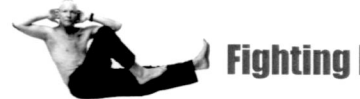 **Fighting Fit Abs** - Battle Proven Exercises

He continues to train every day and believes that "you are only as good as your last training session." He still teaches martial arts, self defense and all aspects of bodyweight conditioning personally via his books, CD's, DVD's and seminars to people who want to change their lives for the better.

Martin has taught his Fighting Fit and Unarmed Combat training program to many British Army Units and he designed it to aid already highly trained and physically fit military troops to propel them to even higher levels of battle readiness and combat fitness. He has taught students from mixed martial arts, kickboxing, shotokan, Wado, men and women's self defense and many more over the years and his ongoing mission is to "help people from all far corners of the World to lead a healthy, safe and successful life."

INTRODUCTION

I have always been interested in fitness, strength, flexibility and realistic training methods and when I think back to over thirty combined years in the British Army and Martial Arts I have learned a lot. The great thing is that I am passing this on to you in this book like I have done in my International best seller Secrets of Fighting Fit Exposed, Battle Proven Exercises for Strength, Flexibility and Fitness.

When I was an Army Physical Training Instructor at recruit training depot in England a long time ago, a civilian administrative assistant who worked in the Headquarters there, came to me for personal training. Fred was aged about 55 if I remember correctly and although he was powerfully built with a large chest and big arms, he had a massive belly that he had enough of carrying around. He made the decision to do something about it. The other thing was that although his stomach was large it was solid so he did have some muscles there.

I set him on a military exercise program that consisted of running with weight on his back, weight training, swimming and abs exercises along with a dose of exercising in the sauna and, here's the other part of the jigsaw – I placed him on a diet that didn't contain any rogue and unnatural foods. The results were amazing; he lost his belly and could at last see his feet when he looked down.

Fred lost at least 12 inches around his waist and dropped from 16 stones to just over 12 stones and all of that took place in only four months, not bad for a 55 year old!

He achieved more than anybody much younger could do...if they only had 10 percent of Fred's determination......

Now here's the thing – can you do the same as Fred?

No question about it YES you CAN! and even more so as I have moved on since then with even more effective training methods of which you will soon be learning about later on in this book.

Now, I know that you have made a big commitment in purchasing this book and I congratulate you on doing so, but let me say straight away that you are going to have to train very hard to build your abs and mid section – there is no quick fix, you have to give a lot of sweat and get a bit of pain to get where you want to be. Some of you may get a 'six pack' some of you may not; it doesn't matter either way as you are going to achieve a physically functional and powerful body as long as you make the mental commitment to go for it and to not give up like most people unfortunately do.

If (when) you do make the commitment to get into awesome, lean mean shape and start following the exercises I am going to show you, then I guarantee that your body will completely change; your entire mid section will become very strong along with your internal organs, lower back and hip flexors. No isolation exercises here, I'm

 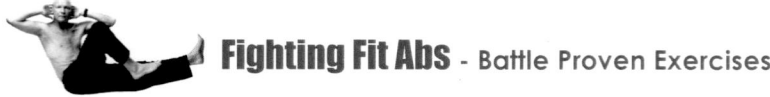

talking functional and conditioned strength along with life prolonging good overall health. This is my aim – to show you how to develop a strong functional mid section and body that others will envy....

Straight into it then and I want you to make a promise to yourself that you will do my exercises each and EVERY morning immediately after you get out of bed. I also want you to pay strict attention to your breathing – how are you breathing now? You see, many people, in fact I do believe the majority of the population either training or sedentary do not breathe correctly, they only take shallow, weak breaths – this achieves zilch; it does nothing to improve the function and health of your internal organs and it won't help you shrink your waistline.

When you breathe strong from your abdomen it makes your entire mid section stronger and more powerful and revitalises all of your internal organs. Oxygen is there to be used so breathe strong and deep and also hold your breath as you feel your chest expand and your stomach contract and then tense your abs at the same time.

If you want to win your battle to burn the flab off from around your waist, then this is what you have to do.

I'll finish by asking you to not just read this book but to do the exercises contained within and transform your body and your life forever.

"Taking the first step is what separates the winners from the losers. Don't be a loser."

VERY IMPORTANT:

Go to my website at **www.MartinDayFitness.com** and provide me with your name and e-mail address so that I can send you a FREE fitness, health, motivation and training tip EVERY week. I promise to keep you positive, determined, informed and inspired. You won't believe how great they are until you get them so don't lose out. If you are serious about the "new you" that is, so don't delay, do it today.

CONTENTS

STARTING TIPS AND INSTRUCTIONS

Have a determined positive attitude
Visualize what you want to achieve
Write down your goals and refer to them every day
Don't just 'exercise' the mid section – work your internal organs also
Focus your mind like a laser on what you are doing
Train your body as a whole and not in isolation
Focus your mind from the inside out – squeeze and tighten
Concentrate on deep breathing
Concentrate on the health benefits that you are achieving
Train every day
Eat only natural foods (most of the time)
Don't make excuses not to train
Don't give up
Don't be lazy

Remember: You don't need any equipment – the exercises can be done anywhere and it won't cost you anything! How about that as an added incentive to get started?

YOU'LL GET FAT IF YOU MAKE EXCUSES

I'm sure you know who they are, the overweight people who can't exercise, can't get out of bed early, can't push themselves hard today, can't change to healthy foods yet, can't get motivated, feel ill all the time....

It's these excuses that are stopping them losing weight, losing fat and losing the chance to be healthy and invigorated.

If you want to change your life and make a difference then all you have to do is stop making excuses and change the way you think from negative to positive.

**"Great things are achieved by a number
of small things brought together."**

MY FIGHTING FIT FAT LOSS STRATEGY

I had been serving in the British Army for some time when a senior Sergeant gave me the following advice, "Martin, if you want results, if you want to discard fat, feel great, live a long healthy life and prevent disease invading your body; then you MUST eat healthy foods".

Well, you're probably thinking that it's easy to say this, but the bottom line is that in a lot of cases it's not easy to do, you see, it all depends on what YOU want to achieve; it's all about your goals and your future not anyone else's.

It's all about YOU.

I can't do it for you.....

What Do You Do?

Don't eat (or at least cut down) on foods that are packaged, processed, preserved or puree, handed to you through your car window or delivered to your front door.

TO GET LEAN YOU NEED TO EAT NATURAL (NATURES) FOODS.

So follow the law of nature and cut out starch and banish fast foods that are high in carbohydrates and high in fat like chips, hot dogs, burgers, pasta, white bread, spaghetti, fried rice, fried eggs....the list goes on. These are major examples of how to get fat and flabby.

Have you seen the obese quantities of junk food that fat people eat? I see them day in day out and want to shout at them to stop because they are HUGE and they moan that they can't lose weight. Don't be one of them and don't make excuses because you are what you eat and if you eat healthily and exercise every day then you become a REAL person both physically and mentally.

Need I say more?

"The elevator to achieving success is out of order: You will just have to use the stairs one step at a time."

TIPS FOR HEALTHY EATING (NATURES LAW)

1   Cut out foods that contain sugar – especially soft drinks
2   Banish foods that contain salt, chemicals, preservatives
3   Drink lots more water
4   Don't snack if you are inactive
5   Avoid foods that are packaged in bags, boxes or wrappers
6   Don't eat before going to sleep
7   Don't combine natural foods with starches
8   Do snack on healthy foods like fruit, yoghurt and small quantities of nuts

Try and stick to the above as best you can or at least 90% of the time, just bear in mind that you need to let yourself go now and again and eat some 'treats', after all we are only human aren't we?

Fat Storing Foods to Avoid (most of the time)

Fatty, processed meats
Diet drinks – they contain huge quantities of chemicals
Fruit juices – too much sugar
Alcohol
Soft drinks – too much sugar
Butter and margarine
Pancakes, French toast
Cereals
Potatoes – especially chips
Ice cream
Pizza and pasta
White rice
Chocolate
Donuts, muffins, cakes and pastries

By having the discipline to adhere to this I guarantee that you will get lean and shed that flab.

Don't Get Diabetes!

Research shows that people who eat five or more portions per week of processed meat like burgers, hot dogs, bacon, luncheon meat and other similar foods have a 42% increased risk of getting diabetes compared to those who ate less than one portion per week.

Dear Friend,

I left my laptop behind and treated myself to a break from the techie world whilst I focused on running training courses for my students in Perth, Western Australia. It was also great to catch up with dear friends that I hadn't seen for about 6 months as well.

This is what we have been doing:

Patricia & I Left Brisbane on a midday flight with Qantas after a delay of about 40 minutes
at the airport and then a technical problem on the aircraft meant that we had to remain on the plane waiting to take off for another 30 mins whilst this problem was being rectified by their engineers. What's happening with 'the spirit of Australia' these days - they have been having lots of problems which you have probably read or watched on the news?

Anyways, take off no problems and we settled down to a relaxing flight with me going through what I was going to teach in Perth in the way of fitness, strength, flexibility, tournament techniques and self defense. Also watched a great film called The Bank Job with Jason Statham and other great actors.... the Brits can still make great films can't they?

Time for food and we unlocked the tables and ensured our seats were upright which I suppose is what is meant to happen...Got our meal served and.....just as we started tucking into it the bloke that was sat in front of Patricia suddenly catapulted his seat back whilst she was eating her meal.

The result of this was that she couldn't eat it properly because of the lack of space that Mr Ignorant had caused. Time for me to step in, politely of course, ensuring that what I was about to say would ALWAYS avoid potential conflict. I tapped Mr Ignorant on the shoulder and said "excuse me mate but could you pull your seat forward so that Patricia can enjoy her meal as she is getting squashed".

By the way, in case you are wondering, Patricia is not a large woman - she's in great shape (she works out with my Fighting Fit exercises every day like me!). This guy turns round to look at me and gave me the biggest look of disgust and contempt that I have ever seen – man, he had an attitude!But, he did put his seat forward...then even more fun started - his wife looked at Mr Ignorant with a snarl and said something to him that I couldn't hear and proceeded to put her seat back towards me and then catapulted her (large) bodyweight into the seat as many times as she could to cause me aggro.

You see, I am over 6ft 2inches tall and my knees were on the receiving end of the 'blows' of this woman.

What would you have done?

I refused to react to her childish behaviour and smiled at the thought that this couple were going nowhere in life with that kind of attitude. There must have been something seriously wrong with them...I didn't react even though my ego wanted me to do something!

What I tell my students to do is to avoid confrontation – it wasn't as though my life was in danger - although that is a completely different ball game!

Just glad that I know how to defend myself both verbally and physically - go and check out my self defense solutions here and you will see what I mean.

http://www.martindayfitness.com/UnarmedCombat.html

I was of course very aware in case they decided to 'have a go' when we arrived in Perth?

They didn't.

The moral of the story is that you can walk tall and with confidence when you know you are capable of dealing with 'situations' and you don't let your ego get in the way!

Enough said.

Take it easy out there and be aware - but most of all enjoy yourself and don't let other people try and drag you down to their level.

Til next time, have a great week.

Martin Day

P.S. To find out more about self defense, martial arts and bodyweight conditioning exercises that will develop a 'new you', go to **www.MartinDayFitness.com**

 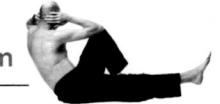

TIPS FOR HEALTHY EATING (NATURES LAW)
CONTINUED...

I'll Be Blunt
The following is what you need to eat if you want to get in shape and it works for me and many others – but don't go berserk on this – life is meant for living so don't forget to treat yourself and have an eating splurge now and again as I do. Go for it for about six weeks and you will see the flab disappear as if by magic and unlike many diet programs where you have to monitor each and every morsel and every calorie that you consume, you don't have to with this so the chances of you staying with it and being successful are much higher than following a 'calorie controlled' diet.

Just follow the law of nature
If you are into sports and you are about to compete or just want to improve your shape, then eat the meals I have listed below.

Lean, Mean Get in Shape Meals
Breakfast - Porridge with skimmed milk or fresh fruit and yoghurt
Mid–Morning - Yoghurt or almonds
Lunch - Tuna salad or roast or baked chicken
Mid–Afternoon - Pear or other fruit
Dinner - Chilli Con Carne or fish with stir fried vegetables

I need to reiterate what I said earlier and that is, every once in a while, say one day a week you treat yourself like I do with maybe chips, chocolate and ice cream and the like as a regular food splurge, but at the same time, don't do it every day or else you'll start to pile on excess weight in no time.

So plan to treat yourself – it will really help you.
You Will Reap the Benefits In a Big Way!

By following my natural meal plan you will;
1   Get lots more energy
2   Rid yourself of unwanted body fat
3   Maintain muscle tone
4   Dynamite your metabolism – they are all natural protein rich foods

Whilst I'm at it here are some other foods that I advise you to eat:

More Good Protein Choices

Kidney Beans	Peas
Milk (Skimmed)	Tuna (canned)
Baked Beans	Mushrooms
Fish (grilled)	Avocado
Beef (lean cut)	Salmon (canned)
Yoghurt	Eggs
Almonds	

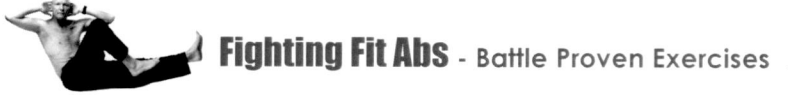

These will DEFINITELY help you to get into the best shape of your life so just take that leap of faith and GO FOR IT.

A word on the benefits of breathing correctly next......

"The road to success is there for the taking, all you must do is to take massive, determined and focussed action."

Better Breathing – Breathe For Life

As you are reading this, I want you to concentrate about HOW you are breathing. Are you breathing shallow and weak or are you breathing strongly from the abdomen and filling your lungs ....believe me, most people breathe shallow and weak from the mouth – this is a worldwide epidemic but you have the opportunity to change – and I want you to change NOW.

I cannot emphasize this enough, you see, by not properly inhaling and exhaling, all the toxins stay in your body so you MUST fully breathe out. The fact is that by holding all these deadly poisons and toxins in your body and not breathing in enough of our life source. Our lungs are heavily contaminated and polluted. It also leads to emotional problems, fear, worry, anxiety and self doubt. Did you know that our bodies are designed to eliminate 70% of its toxins via the lungs? Only 30% of the junk is designed to be eliminated through the skin, bladder, liver and intestines. That's 70% through the lungs!

And of course your lungs are the key to oxygenating your whole body. And when your organs, brain and heart are oxygenated you function better both physically, mentally and emotionally.

REMEMBER

Breathing better will oxygenate your body
Breathing better will help you lose weight
Breathing better will help you eliminate toxins
Breathing better will help you sleep better
Breathing better will improve your sex life
Breathing better will energize you throughout the day
Breathing better will calm you down and lower your heart rate
Breathing better will keep you healthy and help you live longer

Get Breathing!

If you cannot hear your breath whilst you train you're not working hard enough...so get a move on! Studies have shown that when you can hear yourself breathing hard during exercise, it equates to about 65% of your maximum heart rate. This is the minimum level needed for burning fat as fuel during exercise.

Belly Fat Hinders Breathing!

Fat hanging around your stomach makes for shortness of breath during exercise – wads of fat means the body requires more oxygen.

 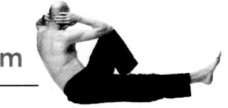

HOW I DISCOVERED THE SECRET TO A FLAT STOMACH

In 1981 I was stationed in Germany and to get straight to the point; I discovered a little known secret method of getting rid of a fat belly and transforming a persons mid section into sheets of steel so that it could withstand punches, kicks and other types of impact.

Well, I eventually mastered this method and used it to great effect many times. I demonstrated and taught it to my soldiers and later on to my martial arts students.

This is how I proved that this training method worked. I got my men together and organised to take them on battle PT and unarmed combat training and called out the biggest soldier to demonstrate on me so that I could prove what could be achieved with a positive mind and a steel hard impact proof body. I ordered him to punch, kick or use a rifle butt to strike me in the stomach. He hesitated at first but did it; quite a few times; he obviously enjoyed assaulting his boss! The amazing thing is that he wasn't able to move or damage me because I had trained myself to withstand his savage blows with the method I will be explaining shortly.

If I can do it so can you. How did I learn how to do this – what was this secret method that was handed down to Joe?

Well I bumped into Joe, who was an 'old sweat' (a soldier that had been in the Army for a long time) in the NAAFI canteen and we started talking about training.

Eventually Joe said that he had learned a supremely effective method of core stomach conditioning that had been passed down to him from his Grandfather. It dated back to the early 1900's.

This was the era of the 'natural' sportsman – they didn't use gym equipment; they used their own bodyweight and were in superb functional condition. They trained their whole body – no isolation exercises were used as they said and proved that it didn't make them as powerful and strong as training the body as a complete unit.

My point exactly – but I didn't know that at the time!

Joe really had my attention as what he was saying made a lot of sense and he was in superb shape....Then he told me the BIG secret and that is to BREATHE DEEP and HOLD YOUR BREATH.
I show you in detail about what to do in my COMBAT DELTA BELLY FLATTENER.

You see, when most people train their mid section' they usually only target one abdominal muscle group, but this method incorporates two other major muscle groups, namely the internal oblique's and the transversus abdominus.

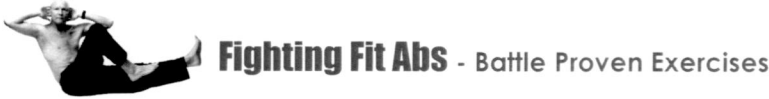

Fighting Fit Abs - Battle Proven Exercises

I, and the people I have taught swear by the method that Joe taught me all those years ago and I'm not exaggerating when I tell you that when you do it, within just a few days you will notice and feel a huge difference in yourself.

Your mid section will feel powerful and hard and you will be walking with a confidence that you have never experienced before – what a revelation!

This exercise really excites me and I am sure that it will for you....at last you will be able to command a flat, strong and powerful stomach without cheating and holding it in – it will happen automatically for you now. This is what building these major muscle groups and your internal organs will do for you.

So here we go – you should be ready to start right now!

"The difference between the impossible and the possible lies in a person's determination."

DON'T WAIT FOR THE NEW YOU

Dear Friend,

In case you aren't aware, time is moving on and really fast - and it could be your last chance to change yourself - to be a new you.

We all have the opportunity, every day in fact, to change to a life of improved health, confidence and peace of mind. Many refuse to change - why?

The way I see it, when you agree to a better life it is ultimately the only way- but why are some people afraid of it?

It's because it needs a shift from your comfort zone based on your current lifestyle, your job, your social life and the way you think and much more.

Your comfort zone is a terrible thing because it's always easier, but dangerous to keep with the familiar than slide into a better life.

When you make the decision to travel in a new direction, it will assist you to get rid of the aggro, the dramas and bring forth powerful energy, health and success into your life.

To that end I have arranged to help you move to this positive level in an easy way.

I give away my best selling books Secrets of Fighting Fit Exposed and Defend Yourself! Ketsugo as gifts along with my Army Special Forces Workouts and Ultimate Flexibility training DVD - all at no cost to you when you go for my Fighting Fit book and DVD pack!

The only thing that I want you to do to get them is to make the decision to lead a better life.

Don't block the positive energy from supercharging your life.

Take it from me it takes a special person with courage, confidence and determination to go for what you really want to happen.

Well, when are you going to get the courage, determination and confidence to grab what you really want?

Why not do it today. Just go here to start: **www.MartinDayFitness.com**
Martin Day

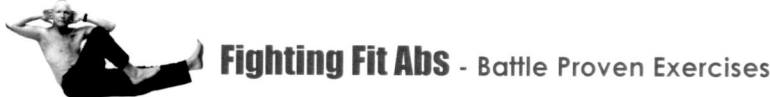

THE HIT LIST

The Hit List (at least three of them) must be done each and every day ideally as soon as you get out of bed, just make sure that your stomach is completely empty. By carrying out these exercises straight away you will set yourself up for the day with lots of energy and it will also help your internal organs, circulation and digestive system to function correctly.

These exercises will also ensure that you get stronger, fitter, flexible and have more stamina, concentrating in the main on your abdominal, oblique and lower back muscles.

It's vitally important when training your mid section that you focus your mind on everything that is involved when carrying out the exercises - and not just your abs. To do isolation exercises is wrong – the KEY to real results is to train ALL the muscles associated with your abs, like your lower back and hip flexors. For all of you that train in martial arts and other combat sports, you will know that your body needs to be conditioned as a complete entity and not broken down into isolated muscle groups.

If you are short of time or just want a focused blast then go for the Hit List – these eight battle proven exercises really work and you will feel and see the results FAST.

"Victory belongs to the most persevering"
– Napolean Bonaparte

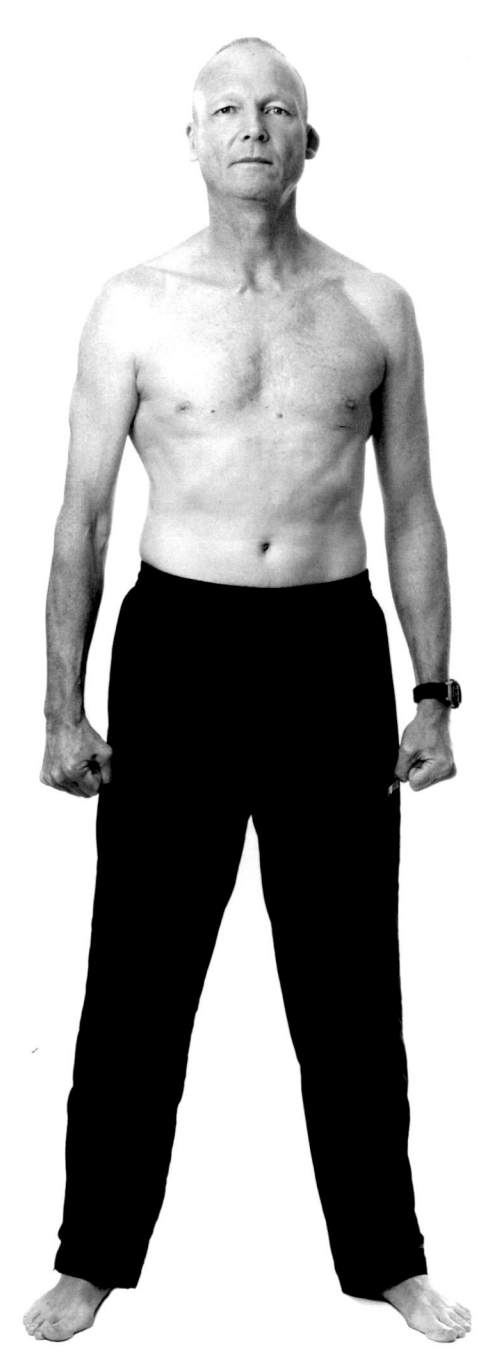

Fighting Fit Abs - Battle Proven Exercises

COMBAT DELTA BELLY FLATTENER

This is what my mate Joe taught me after it had been passed down to him from his Grandfather in the early 1900's; I have utilised my experience and added a few more details so that this exercise is even more effective. Bear in mind also that you are going to work your chest, shoulders, throat, neck and arms. Internal organs also get a workout along with increased blood circulation and this will make you healthier and less prone to illness.

Note: This exercise and all the others should be carried out prior to eating.

1   Stand straight with your feet shoulder feet apart and look forward.

2   Visualise what you want to achieve – think steel hard flat abs.

3   Relax your whole body starting from your head to toes and breathe in deeply through your nose. Make sure that your arms are relaxed and hanging naturally.

4   Inhale about 99% and then take a few more short sharp breaths so that you completely fill your lungs to capacity.

5   As you breathe in, pull your stomach/abdomen in towards your spine. Don't let your stomach expand.

6   Once your lungs are full to the brim, gently close your teeth together and exhale your breath SLOWLY whilst making a 'hissing' sound as your breath passes through your teeth. At the same time squeeze your abdominal muscles as hard as you can – make them steel hard and impact proof!

7   Do this until ALL the air is expelled from your lungs – it helps if you tense your fists as hard as you can so that your stomach muscles and internal organs are hammered into shape atthe same time.

8   By breathing out as hard as you can you will achieve two other important things – firstly, you will take in a large, full amount of fresh air on the next rep, and secondly, you will squeeze the lungs like bellows to get rid of all that stale, old air in there. You might want to have a tissue handy just in case something flies out of you nostrils.

Carry out this exercise for at least five minutes morning, evening and whenever you can – even if you're waiting in a shop queue. Start slowly and then gradually increase the time so that results will be faster.

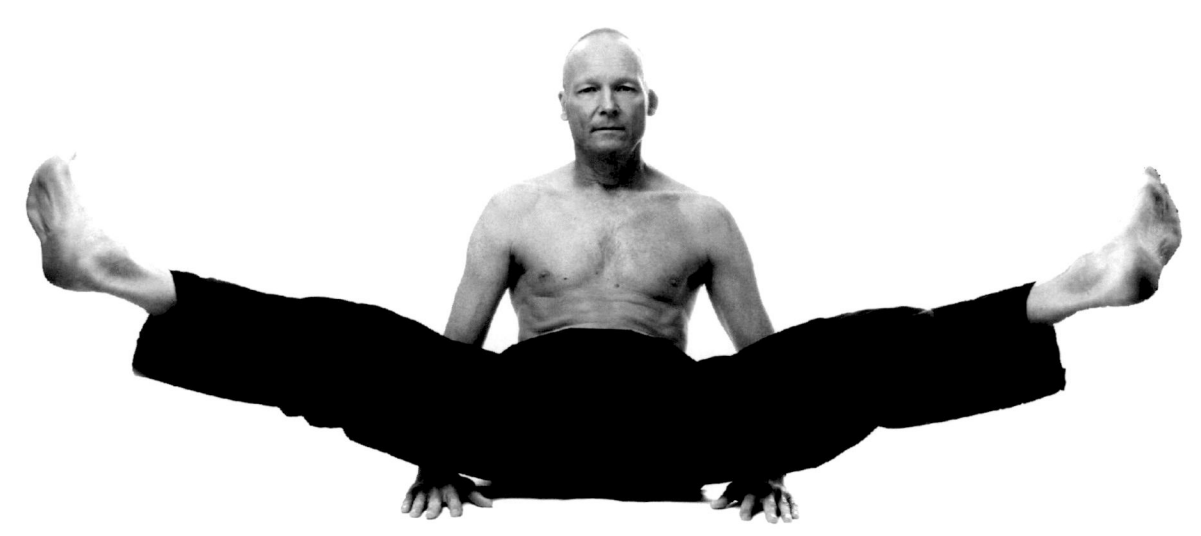

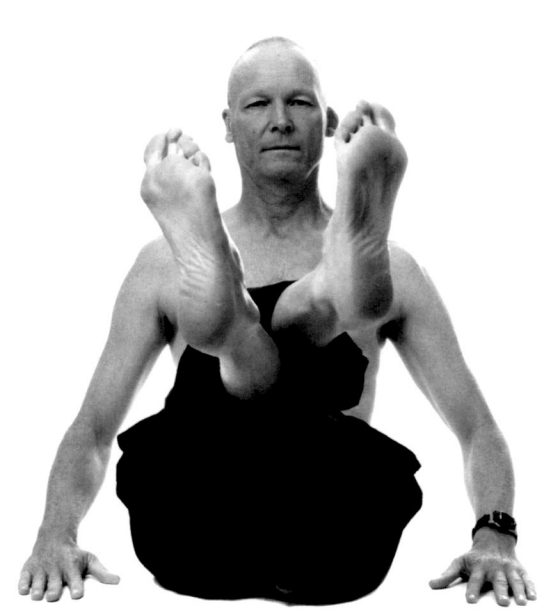

Fighting Fit Abs - Battle Proven Exercises

EXERCISE ALPHA – SCISSORS

This exercise hits your upper and lower abdominals, neck, shoulders, lower back, hip flexors and legs.

1   Get onto your back and place your hands at arms length at your sides.

2   Keep your legs as straight as you can and lift them about six inches off the ground.

3   Concentrate and open your legs as wide as you can and then move them towards each other and cross one over the other in a scissor like motion.

4   Breathe in when you open your legs and breathe out when you cross them. Carry out 25- 50 repetitions and aim for 100 when you get stronger.

VERY IMPORTANT:

Go to my website at **www.MartinDayFitness.com** and provide me with your name and e-mail address so that I can send you a FREE fitness, health, motivation and training tip EVERY week. I promise to keep you positive, determined, informed and inspired. You won't believe how great they are until you get them so don't lose out. If you are serious about the "new you" that is, so don't delay, do it today.

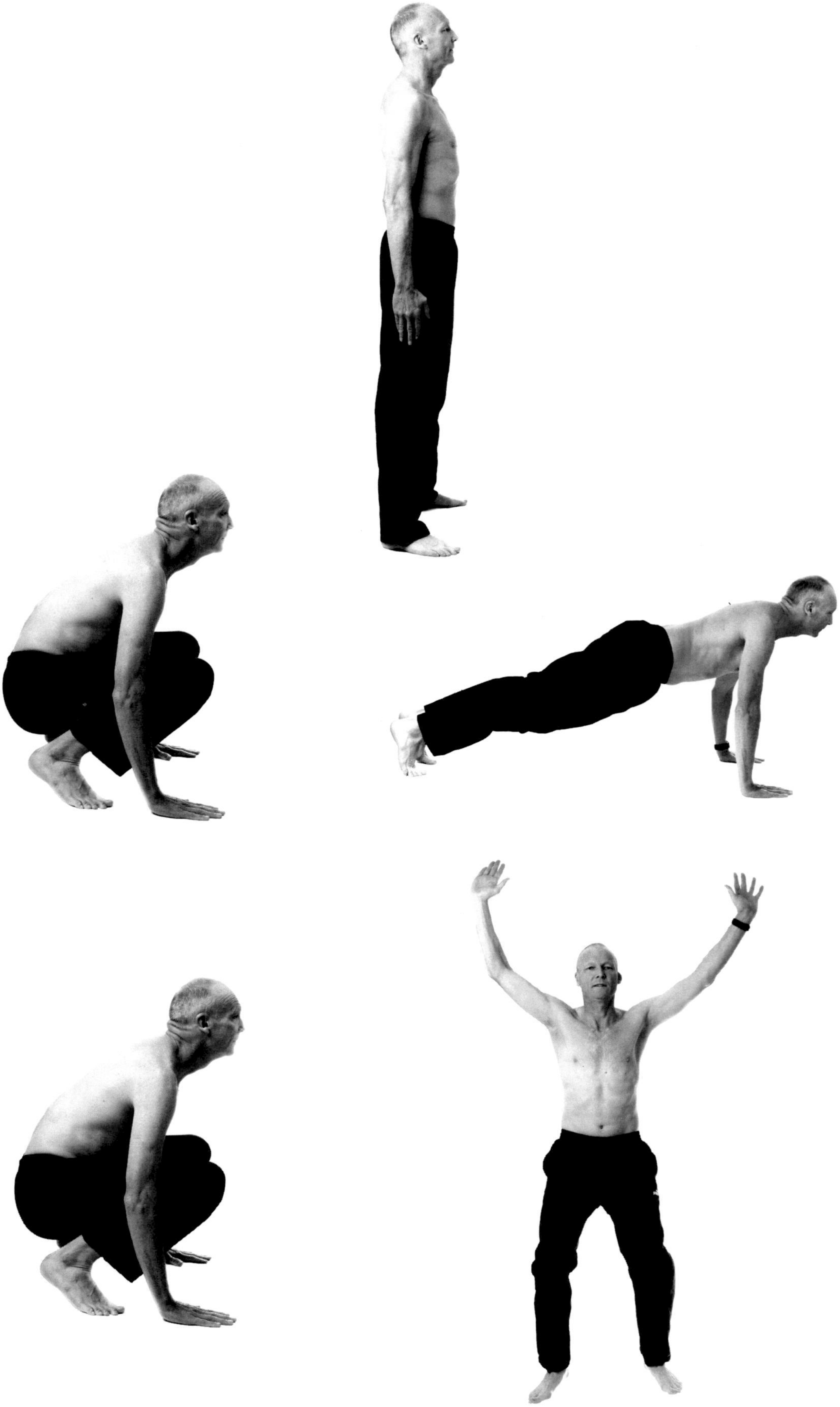

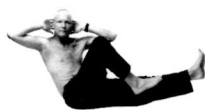 **Fighting Fit Abs** - Battle Proven Exercises

EXERCISE BRAVO – ARMY BURPEES

BURPEES are used to train the British Army and I have taught and practised it myself over many years – I have also included BURPEES in my martial arts training syllabus. It's a superb overall bodyweight conditioning exercise and the deep breathing makes your lungs much stronger.

You will also notice that your abs, legs, arms and hips get a serious hammering.

1   Adopt a standing position with your feet slightly wider than shoulder width apart and ensure your arms are hanging naturally to your sides.

2   Squat down and place your hands in front of your feet.

3   Take your weight on your hands and drive your legs back into a press up position making sure that your back is straight.

4   Drive you legs back into your chest (like a squat thrust).

5   Propel yourself upwards and jump off the ground as high as you can.

6   Carry out a minimum of ten sets and breathe as naturally as you can throughout.

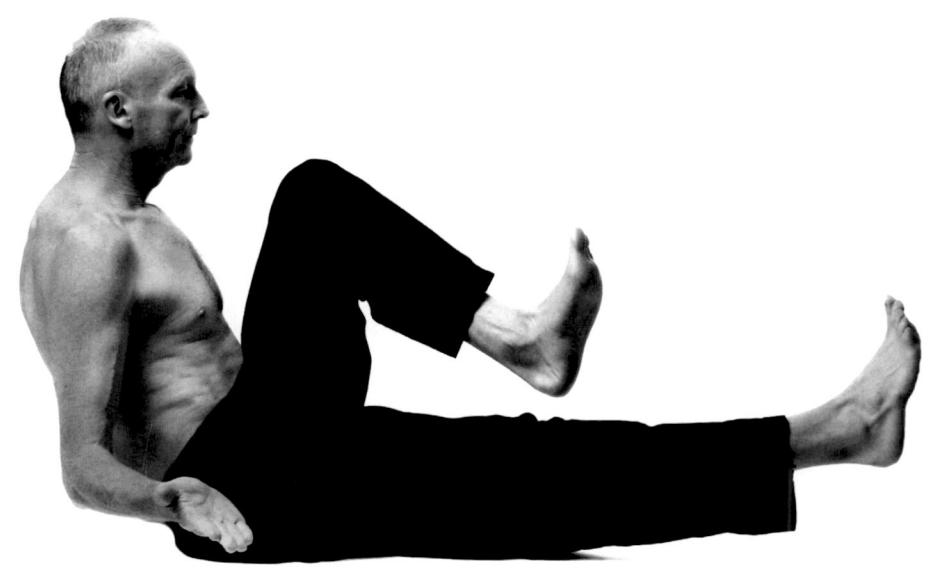

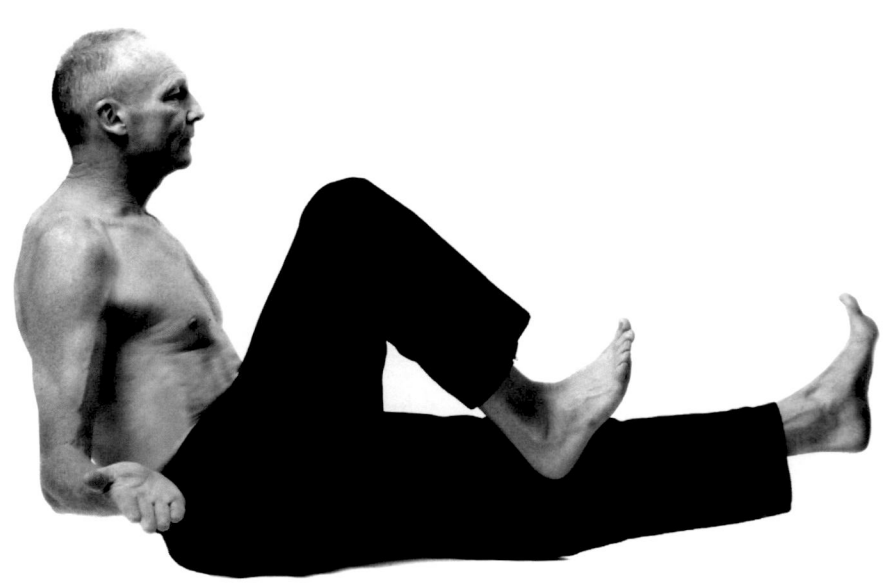

Fighting Fit Abs - Battle Proven Exercises

EXERCISE CHARLIE – HANDS OUT CYCLING

This Hit List exercise will challenge your abdominal muscles in a big way. Additionally, it strengthens your back, hip flexors and legs. The action of holding your arms out will not only assist your balance but will strengthen your upper body.

It improves your leg circulation as well.

1   Sit on the ground and ensure that your shoulders are raised up, keep your legs as straight as you can about six inches off the ground.

2   Draw both knees up to your chest.

3   Balance and keep the tension on your abs and start bicycling whilst positioning your arms outwards, palms open.

4   Keep your back straight, breathe normally and concentrate.

5   Do as many reps as you can.

Note: both legs must remain off the ground throughout this exercise.

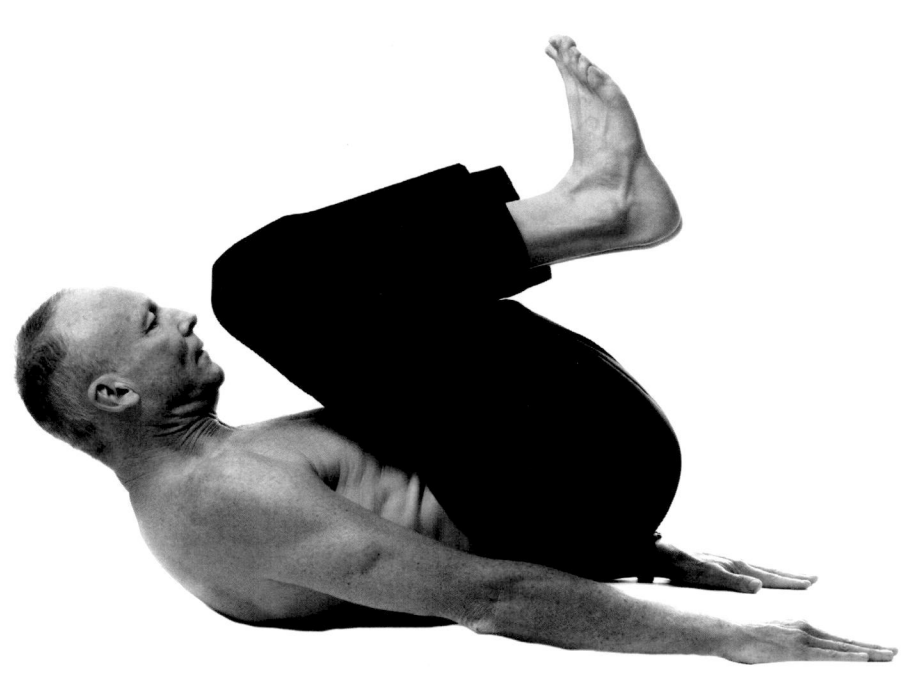

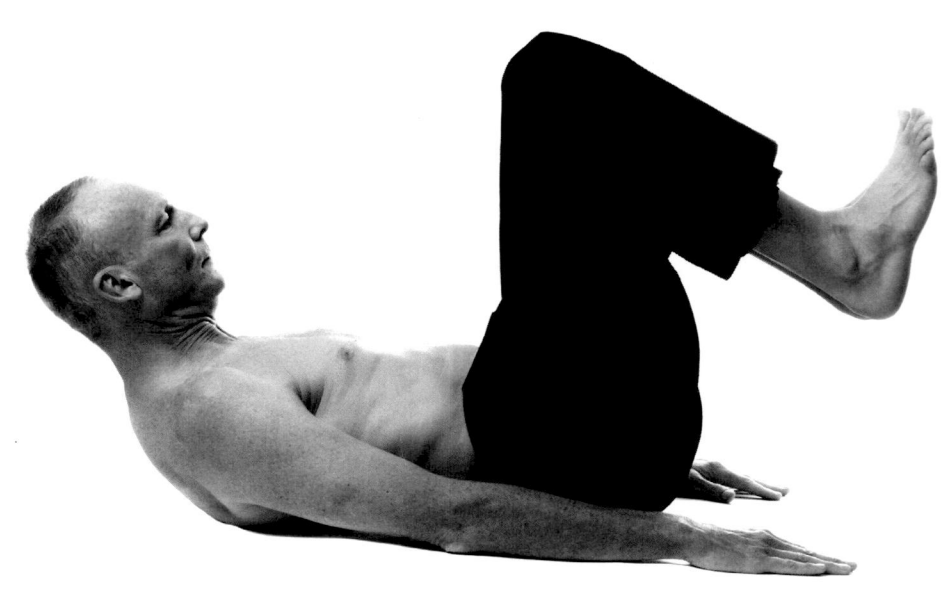

EXERCISE DELTA
KNEES TO CHEST WITH TENSION

Targets your upper and lower abs, lower back and hip flexors and helps your balance and co-ordination and core strength.

1   Adopt a position lying on your back with your legs and arms straight.

2   Look up and keeping your shoulders on the ground, pull your knees in towards your chest.

3   Use your arms for balance and hold your knees to your chest and tense your mid section in an isometric contraction for ten seconds.

4   Relax your knees and mid section and allow your knees to travel about twelve inches so that your upper thighs are at a right angle to the ground and hold for ten seconds.

5   Repeat as many times as you can.

6   Breathe in knees up and breathe out knees down.

Note: this is a hugely effective isometric (tension) exercise and you will notice big gains in your abs strength almost immediately.

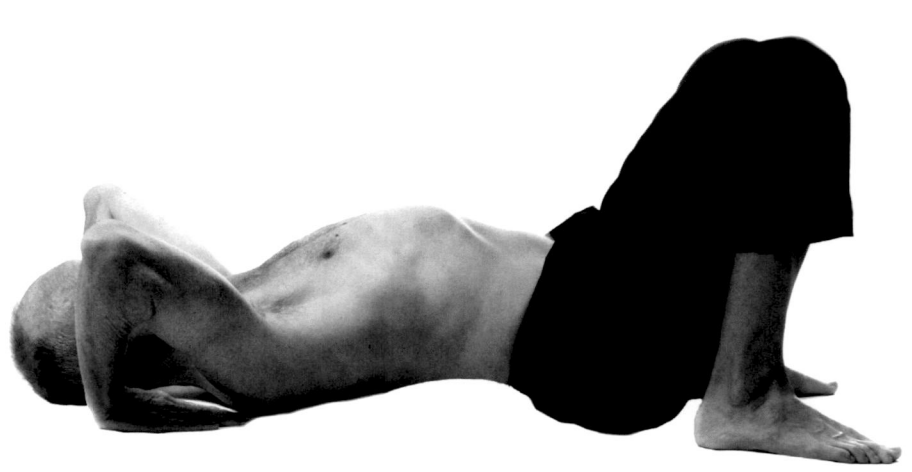

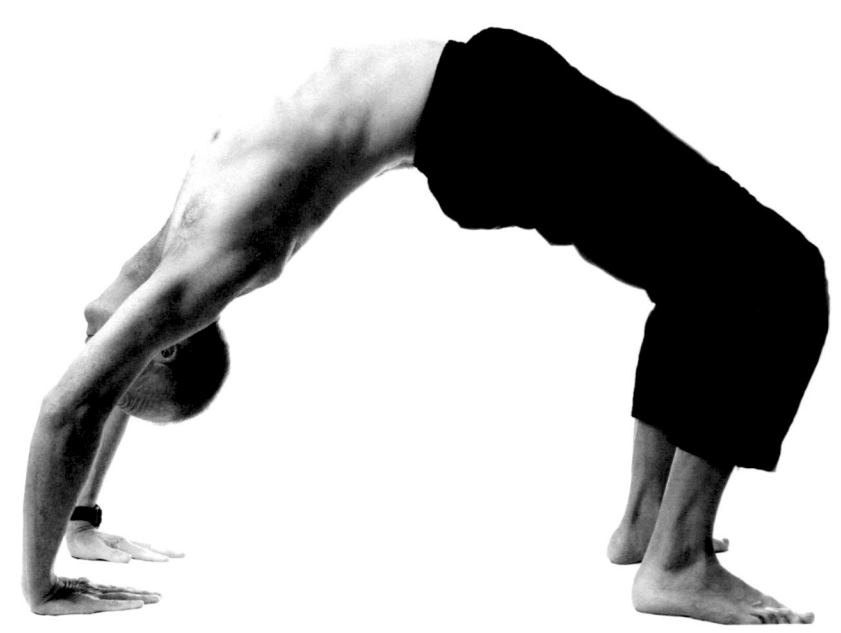

Fighting Fit Abs - Battle Proven Exercises _____

EXERCISE ECHO – BRIDGE

An amazing, all in comprehensive elite exercise that develops strength, power and flexibility throughout your whole body. It targets the neck, back, upper and lower abs, upper shoulders, and improves spinal strength and flexibility; this is particularly important because it prevents common spinal injuries. I have picked up injuries in my neck, shoulders and lower back region and by doing the BRIDGE, I and many others have eliminated the pain and injury. A lot of people find this difficult to believe, but it is TRUE.

Many other people that do the BRIDGE testify that it is a brilliant cure and injury prevention exercise not only for the back, but the neck and shoulders as well. If you find this exercise difficult at first, which you probably will, then just persevere and enjoy it. Don't worry, you will soon be doing the BRIDGE like a pro and reaping the massive health benefits. Start slowly and be careful not to overarch or over twist.

Relax, focus and go:

1   Lie on your back with knees bent, feet or toes on the ground.

2   Position your hands by your shoulders, elbows high.

3   Power up off your legs and arms and position your head back as far as you are able to so that the top of your head is facing towards the floor.

4   Concentrate on arching your back, forcing your chest upwards.

5   Stretch up and rock back and forward, slowly placing as much weight on your head and/or hands as safely as possible.

6   Hold for as long as you are able and breathe!

7   Breathe in when you power upwards and breathe out as you lower yourself to the ground.

8   It's a good idea to get into the bridge 10-20 times before holding it for about 1-3 minutes.

Note: Slow your breathing down as much as you can when holding the BRIDGE.

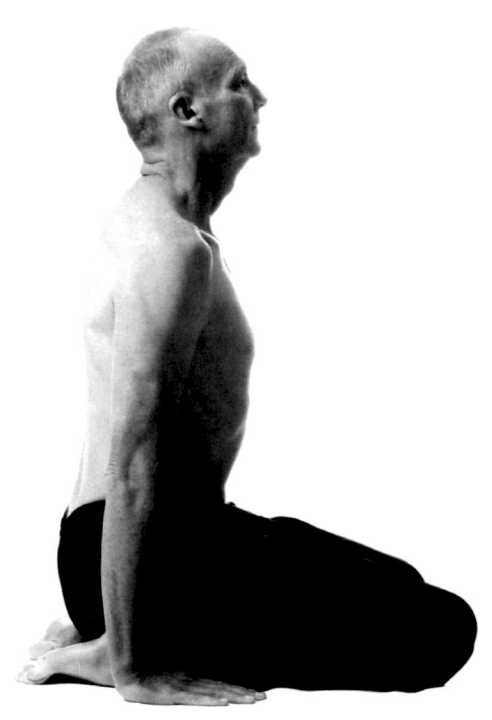

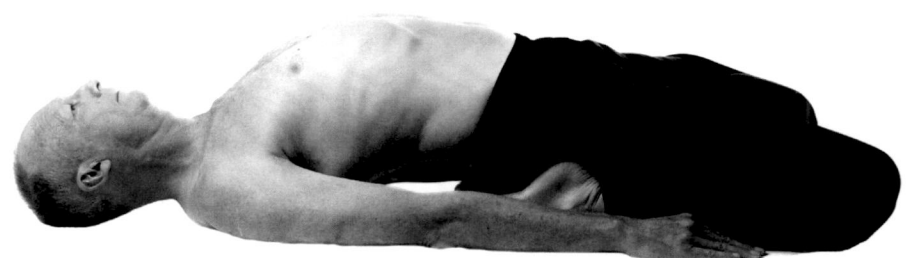

Fighting Fit Abs - Battle Proven Exercises

EXERCISE FOXTROT
– KNEELING STRETCH BACK

Stretch out!

This one really loosens you up and stretches and strengthens your abs, thighs, lower back, ankles, buttocks and hip flexors.

You also get a supercharged workout in your abs when you tense and hold in the fully extended position.

1   Adopt a kneeling position and point your toes towards the floor.

2   Sit on your heels and insteps or with your heels and insteps outside of your legs. Keep your back straight, hips pushed forward and place your hands on the floor.

3   Look up and slowly lower your head to the floor keeping your body straight and tense your abs. You may need to use your hands to support yourself as you go down when you begin this one.

4   Hold your lowest position with your arms parallel to the floor and look up and back. Take five deep breaths.

5   Using your strength and keeping your back straight and hips forward, return to the starting point. Use your hands to support yourself until you get stronger.

6   Open (breathe in) chest down, close (breathe out) chest up.

7   Blast 5 to 20 reps.

Note: Don't go down too far when you first start this exercise!

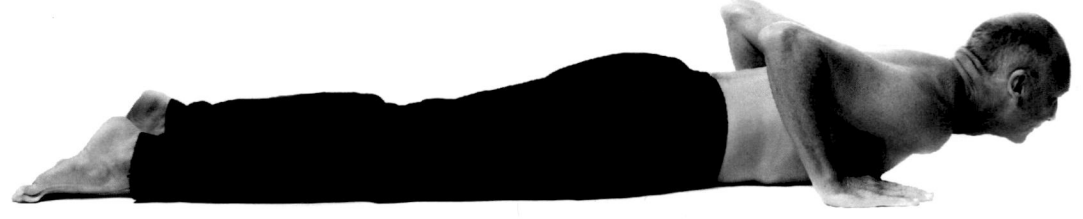

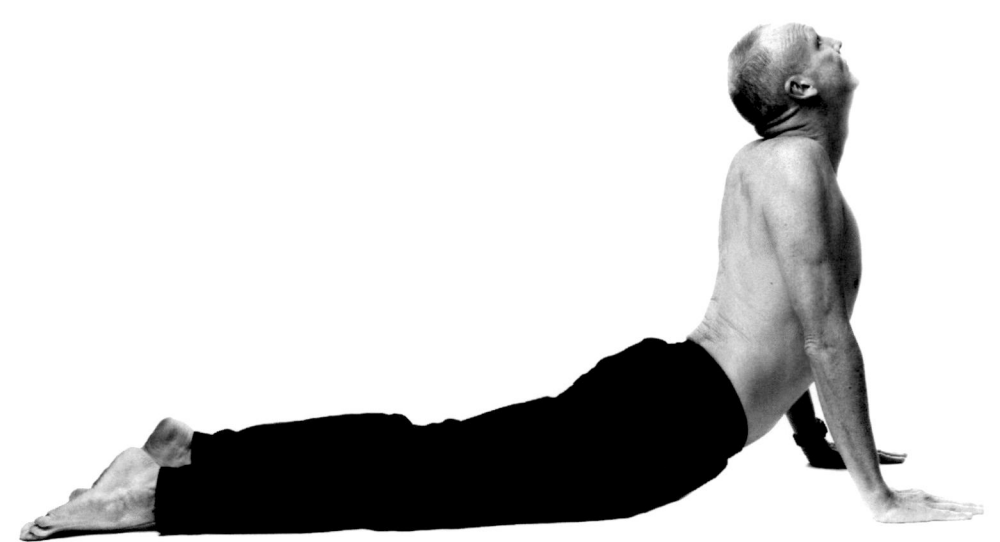

Fighting Fit Abs - Battle Proven Exercises

EXERCISE GOLF - COBRA (PUSH UP CURL)

Really stretches and strengthens your abs, shoulders, neck and your spine. How many people do you see 'stooping' with their shoulders hunched from poor posture?

Poor posture results in health problems – and specifically major back problems. Well, here is the solution; another piece of the jigsaw; just do this exercise, along with the BRIDGE and incorporate some other exercises in this book along with the bodyweight exercises that I teach in my other international best seller Secrets Of Fighting Fit Exposed and you are going to reap the amazing benefit of a strong, healthy spine and more.

1   Get onto the ground face down and place your hands in line with your shoulders with hands facing forward as you would if you were preparing for a press up.

2   Look up and push up with you arms, arching your back as far as you can.

3   Hold this position with your arms straight and your spine bent backwards for a minimum of ten seconds.

4   Repeat 10 -20 times.

5   Breathe in when you power upwards and breathe out as you lower yourself to the ground.

VERY IMPORTANT:

Go to my website at **www.MartinDayFitness.com** and provide me with your name and e-mail address so that I can send you a FREE fitness, health, motivation and training tip EVERY week. I promise to keep you positive, determined, informed and inspired. You won't believe how great they are until you get them so don't lose out. If you are serious about the "new you" that is, so don't delay, do it today.

INTERMEDIATE FIGHTING FIT ABS EXERCISES

The following exercises are designed for the beginner or advanced practitioner to do.

Some of you who have been training regularly and are in reasonable shape will be able to do most of the exercises and the reps I have nominated almost straight away. But to all of you, regardless of what level of fitness and strength levels you are currently at, I want you to concentrate HARD on proper form (technique) and efficient and correct deep breathing.

Then I want you to make sure that you change the sequence of the exercises every time that you train not forgetting, (and this is vitally important) that you carry out the HIT LIST EVERY DAY first thing as this will build your training foundation like building blocks on the way to constructing a house.

When you do the eight exercises in the HIT LIST each morning straight out of bed, what you are in fact doing is resetting your nervous system and conditioning your body for the day ahead and further intensive training later on in the day – your main training workout.

It will also give you a concentrated energy boost for the day and make you feel healthy, loose and ALIVE.

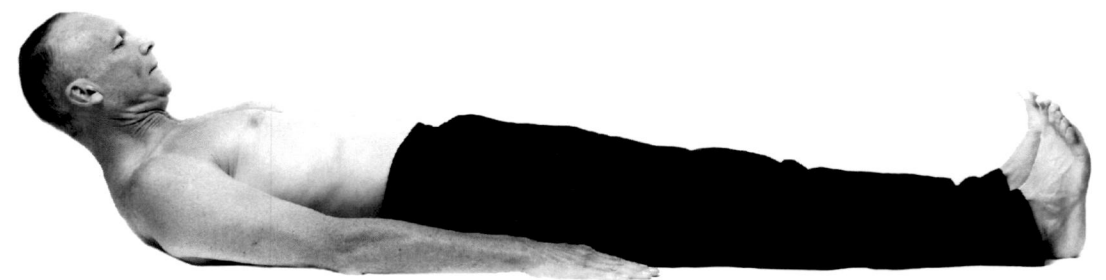

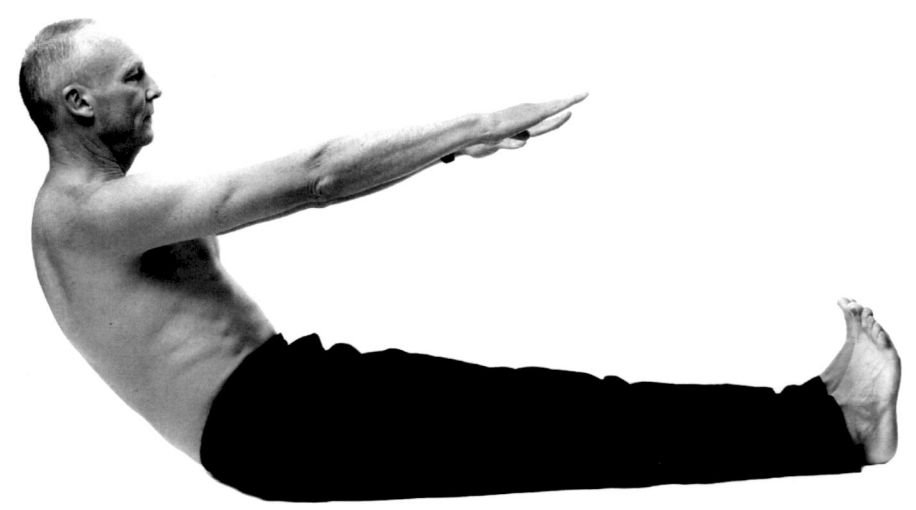

Fighting Fit Abs - Battle Proven Exercises

STRAIGHT LEG CURL UPS

You hit your upper abs and at the same time you will strengthen your lower back and hip flexors with this exercise.

Note: Don't bounce or use any sort of momentum to get yourself off the ground as this is cheating - you are only cheating yourself so just do your best.

1   Lie on your back and ensure that your legs are straight and your arms by your sides.

2   Now, SLOWLY lift your upper body off the ground making sure your legs remain on the ground and straight.

3   Curl your toes back in towards you to get a better hamstring stretch as you lift your body to about a 45 degree angle and reach forward with your arms.

4   Tense and hold for 3-5 seconds and repeat as many times as you can.

5   Breathe in as you lift up and out as you lower yourself down.

Ensure that you do not rest on the floor after each repetition and do not tense your quad muscles (legs) as you are carrying out this exercise – focus on building your abs.

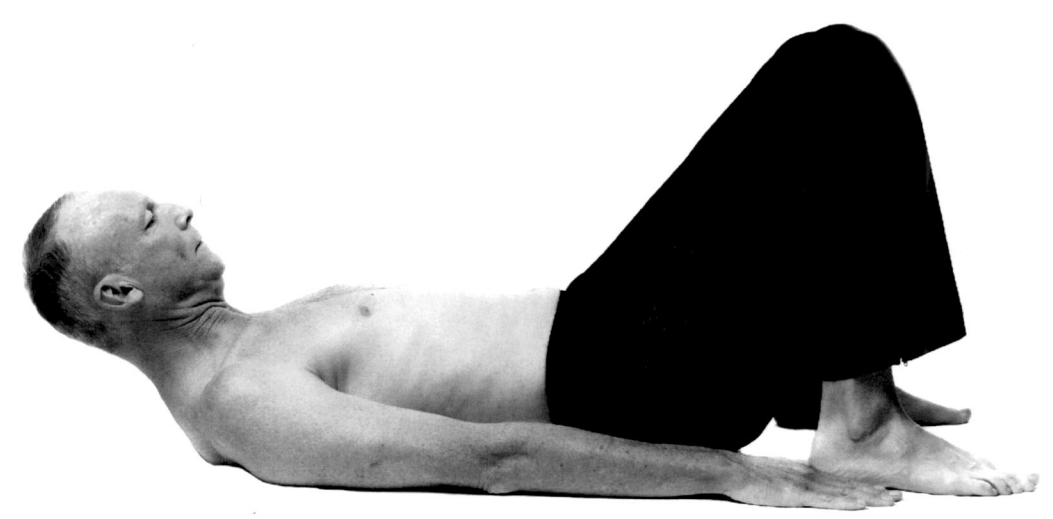

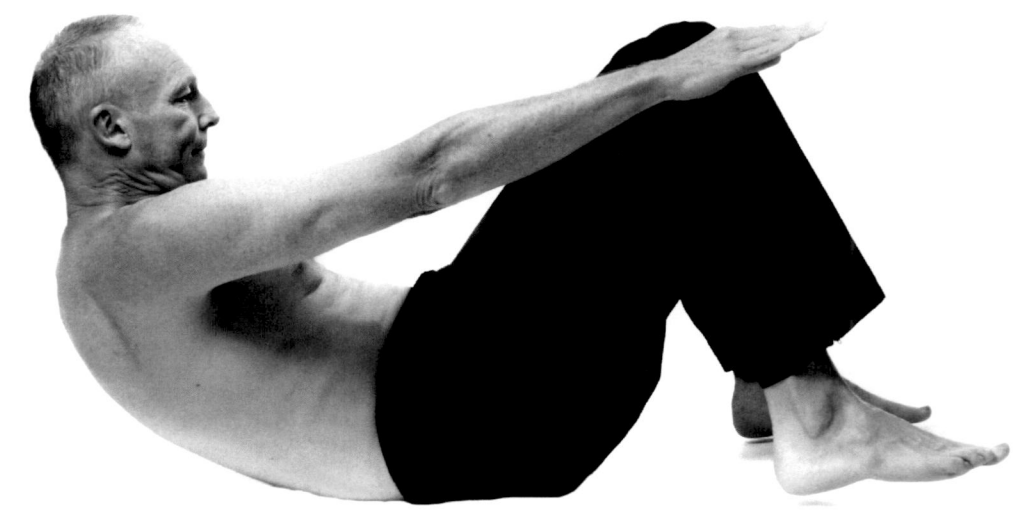

Fighting Fit Abs - Battle Proven Exercises

BENT LEG CURL UPS

A variation of the STRAIGHT LEG CURL UPS and this time it hits your upper and lower abs, lower back and hip flexors. As before, make sure that you don't bounce or use any sort of momentum.

1   Lie on the ground and draw your feet in towards you with arms to your sides and legs bent.

2   Reach forward SLOWLY with your hands pointing to your knees and raise your upper body off the ground to a 45 degree angle.

3   Tense and hold for 3-5 seconds and repeat as many times as you can.

4   Breathe in as you lift up and breathe out as you lower yourself down.

Once again, ensure that you do not rest on the floor after each repetition and do not tense your quad muscles (legs) as you are carrying out this exercise – focus on building your abs.

"There are no secrets to success. It is the result of preparation, hard work and learning from failure." – General Colin Powell

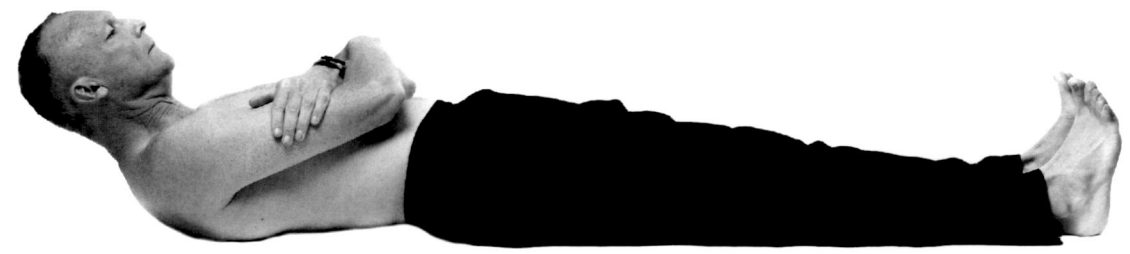

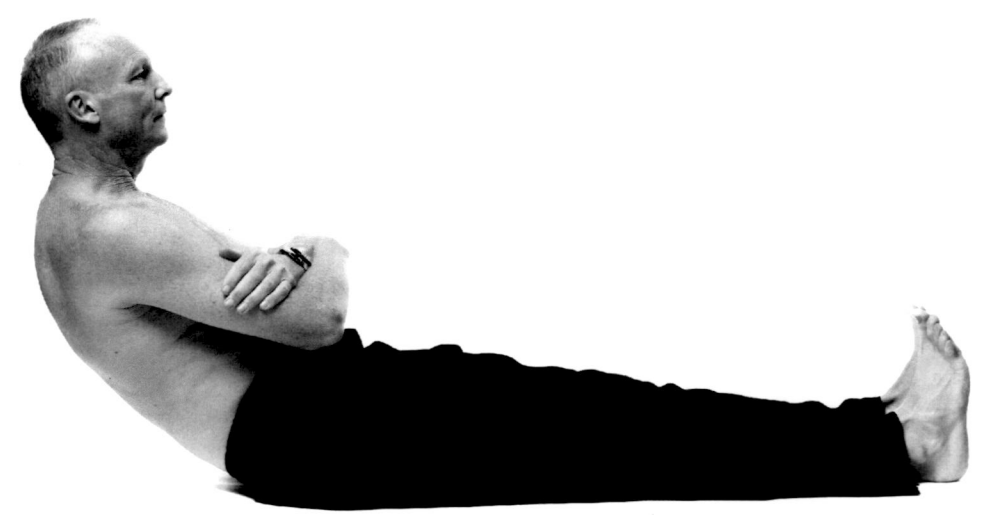

Fighting Fit Abs - Battle Proven Exercises

PREACHER CURL UPS

A good, solid core and abs strengthening exercise that helps to build a stronger lower back and hip flexors.

1   Adopt a position on your back with your legs straight and your arms folded across your chest.

2   Look forward and remembering to keep your legs on the floor and not using momentum, lift up to an angle of 45 degrees and tense and hold for 3-5 seconds.

3   Breathe in as you lift up and breathe out as you lower yourself down.

Keep your arms into your chest throughout this exercise and focus on tensing and building your abs.

Note: Every now and again; reach ALL THE WAY UP so that you stretch your hamstrings and back.

Dear Friend,

In case you aren't aware, time is moving on and really fast - and it could be your last chance to change yourself - to be a new you.

We all have the opportunity, every day in fact, to change to a life of improved health, confidence and peace of mind. Many refuse to change - why?

The way I see it, when you agree to a better life it is ultimately the only way- but why are some people afraid of it?

It's because it needs a shift from your comfort zone based on your current lifestyle, your job, your social life and the way you think and much more.

Your comfort zone is a terrible thing because it's always easier, but dangerous to keep with the familiar than slide into a better life.

When you make the decision to travel in a new direction, it will assist you to get rid of the aggro, the dramas and bring forth powerful energy, health and success into your life.

To that end I have arranged to help you move to this positive level in an easy way.

I give away my best selling books Secrets of Fighting Fit Exposed and Defend Yourself! Ketsugo as gifts along with my Army Special Forces Workouts and Ultimate Flexibility training DVD - all at no cost to you when you go for my Fighting Fit book and DVD pack!

The only thing that I want you to do to get them is to make the decision to lead a better life.

Don't block the positive energy from supercharging your life.

Take it from me it takes a special person with courage, confidence and determination to go for what you really want to happen.

Well, when are you going to get the courage, determination and confidence
to grab what you really want?

Why not do it today.

Just go here to start:

www.MartinDayFitness.com

Martin Day

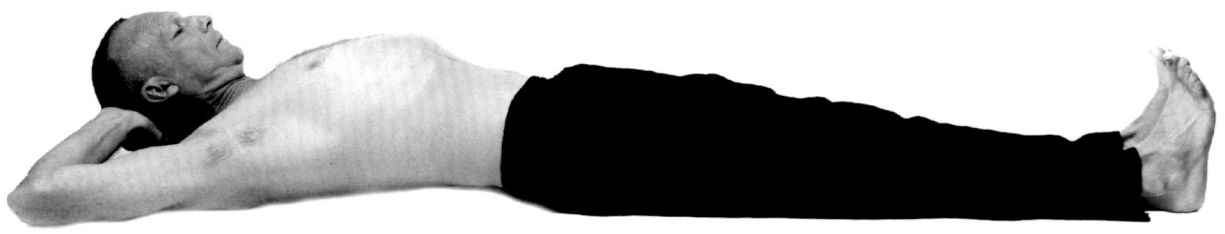

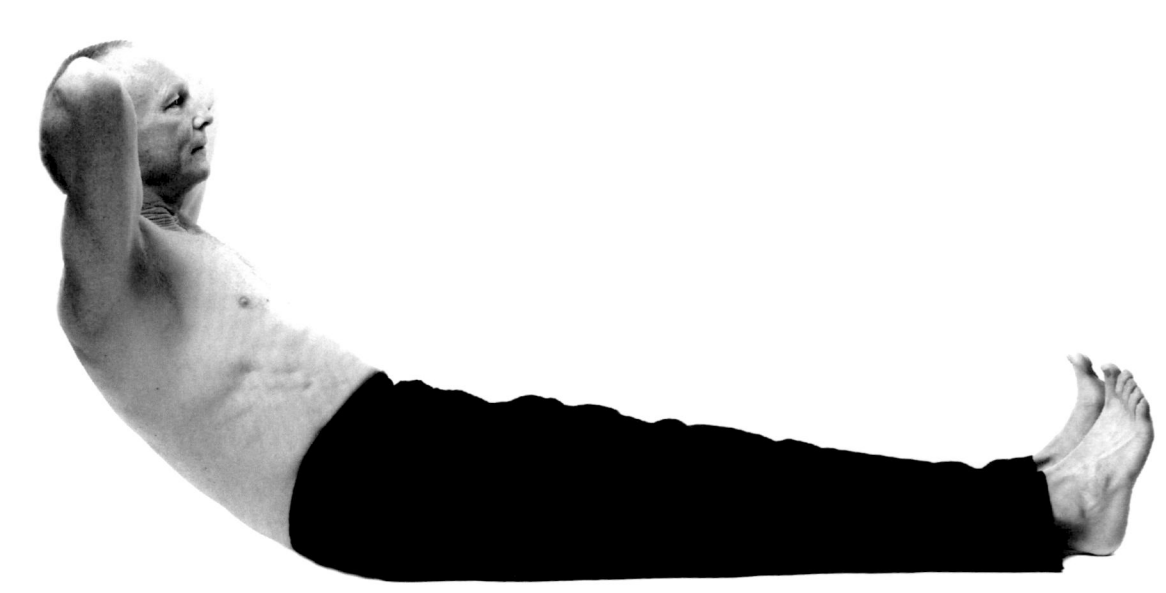

HAMMER CURL UPS

This one is similar to PREACHER CURLS and targets the same muscle groups even more effectively. It is slightly more difficult as your hands are behind your head. Same rules apply as regards momentum, tension and focus.

1   Lie on the ground with your legs straight and your arms by your sides.

2   Place your hands behind your head making sure that your fingers are touching and not clasped.

3   Lift your upper body off the ground SLOWLY and hold at the 45 degree point.

4   Make sure that your legs remain straight and your toes are pulled in towards you and hold the position for 3-5 seconds.

5   Breathe in as you curl up and breathe out as you lower yourself down.

Note: Keep your arms into your chest throughout this exercise and focus on tensing and building your abs.

Every now and again; reach ALL THE WAY UP so that you stretch your hamstrings, back and shoulders.

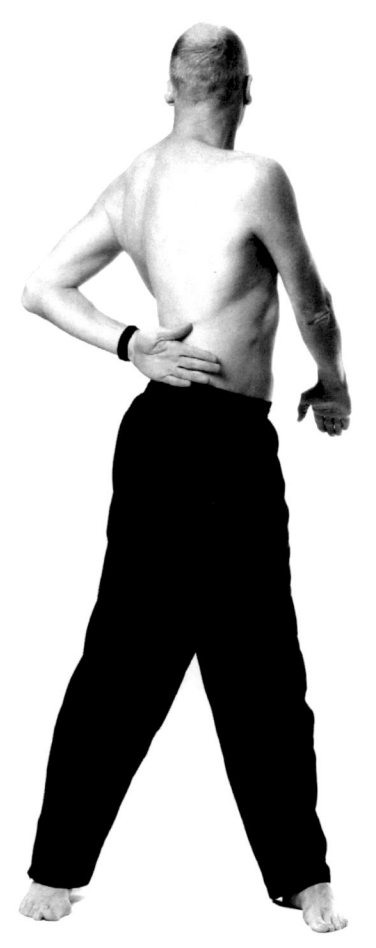

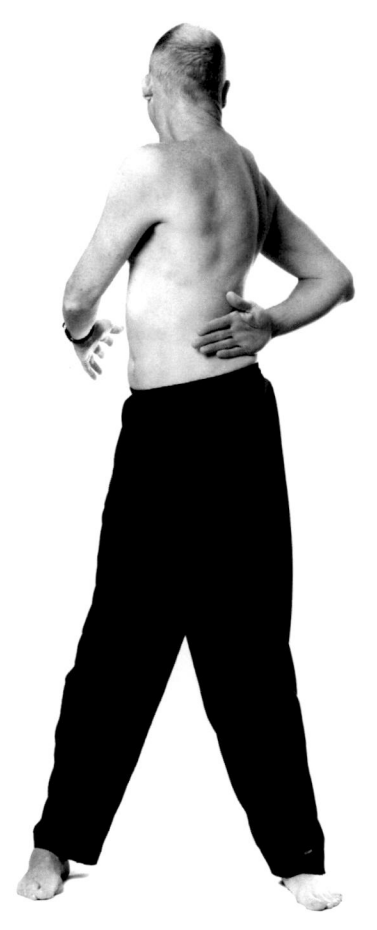

COMBAT KARATE WAIST TWISTS

I teach this drill in my classes as do practitioners of other martial arts systems including Tai Chi and Kung Fu.

It encourages better blood circulation to your internal organs, increases flexibility in your waist and hips and loosens your spine. It also helps to banish back problems and tones your mid section.

1   Stand up straight with your feet slightly wider than shoulder width apart with the whole of your body completely relaxed.

2   Commence turning your upper body from side to side without moving your arms.

3   Keep your feet in exact same position on the ground and let your arms go limp – use centrifugal force to swing your arms from left to right.

4   Twist as far as you are able and at the same time allow your out turned hand to slap your kidney GENTLY. This results in giving your kidneys a massage.

5   Breathe normally as you do this.

6   Carry out 25- 100 reps.

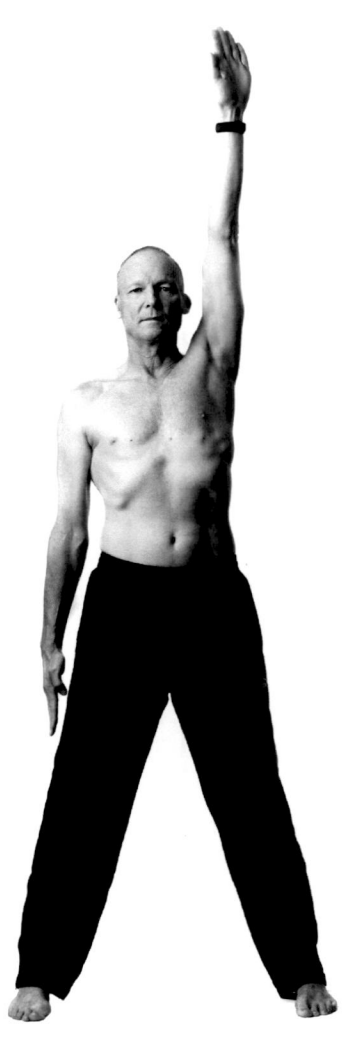

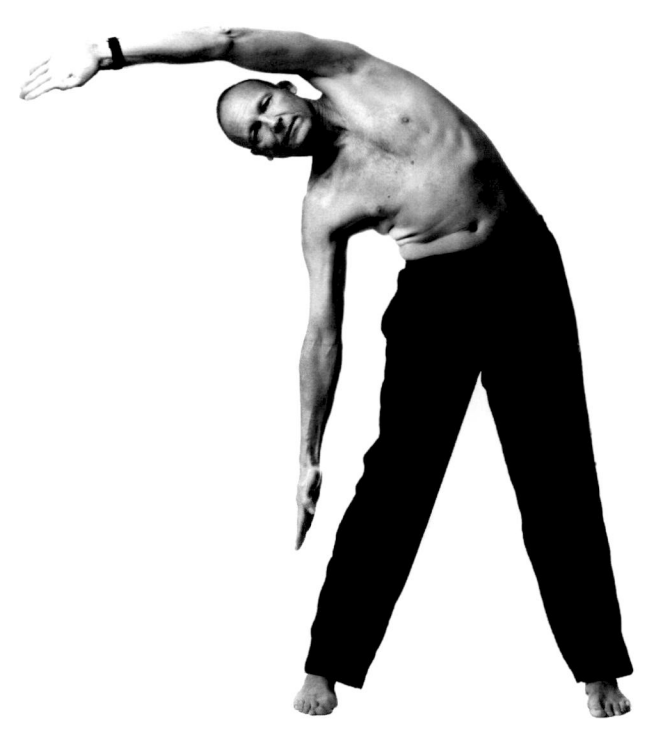

Fighting Fit Abs - Battle Proven Exercises

SIDE REACHES WITH DYNAMIC TENSION

Another great Fighting Fit exercise which helps you to gain strength and enjoy greater flexibility in every direction and tracks in hard on the oblique's (sides of the waist).

1   Stand in a neutral position and ensure that your feet are slightly wider than shoulder-width apart.

2   Reach up as high as you can with your left hand palm turned outwards.

3   Breathe in deeply and stretch down with your right hand towards your right ankle as far as possible and slowly move down and up.

4   Ensure that you do not slump forward as you carry out this dynamic stretch – just move down and up about a couple of inches.

5   Hold this position and stretch with your left hand up and down a few inches twenty to fifty times.

6   Change sides and repeat.

7   Breathe deep when you start each repetition.

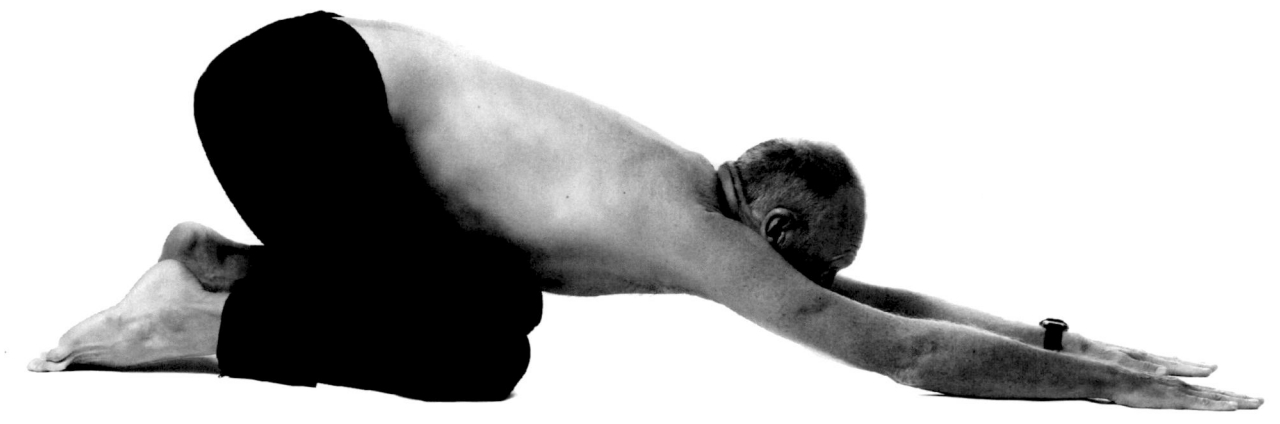

Fighting Fit Abs - Battle Proven Exercises

ISOMETRIC COBRA

This time you are going to strengthen and loosen your spine and at the same time work your abs, chest, shoulders and arms from a different angle.

1   Adopt a kneeling position and then reach out as far forward as you can with your hands, ensuring that your arms are straight.

2   Allow your spine to relax and let gravity do its job.

3   Inhale strongly and then sink your chest down and push your upper body into the ground as hard as you can.

4   Tense your abs strongly whilst breathing out slowly.

5   Hold for 10-30 seconds and relax.

6   Repeat as many times as you can.

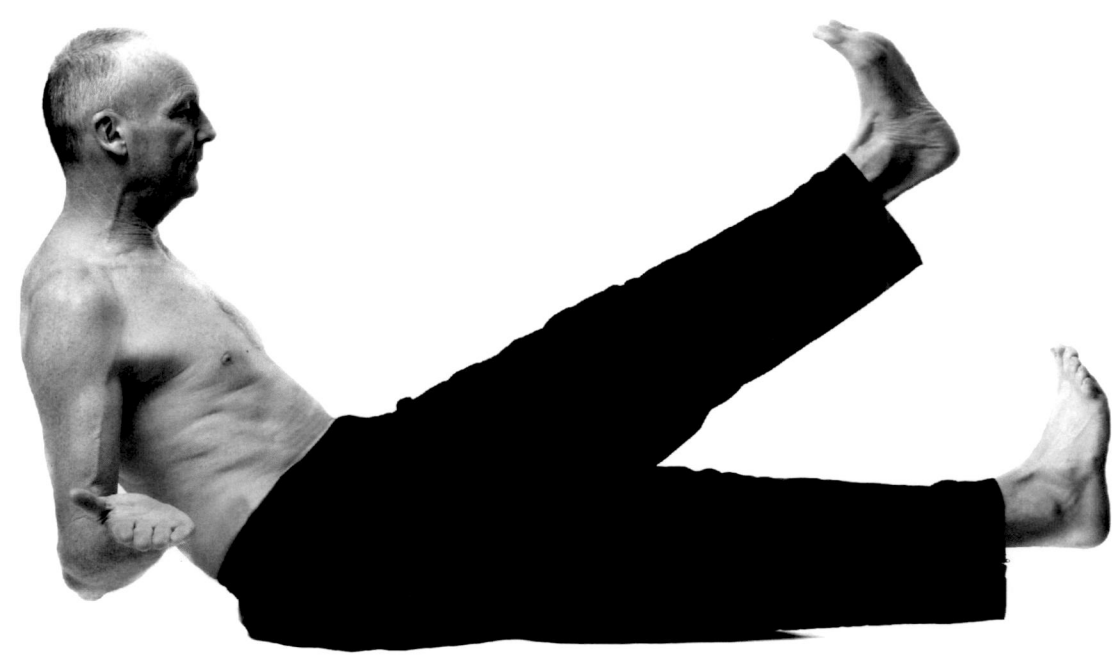

Fighting Fit Abs - Battle Proven Exercises

SWIM KICKS – ARMS OUT

You'll really feel this in your upper abs, hip flexors, lower back and legs. It also helps your balance and co ordination.

1   Lie on your back with legs straight and your arms out slightly bent and with your palms facing up.

2   Look forward towards your feet and then, keeping your legs straight, raise your upper body and legs off the ground, breathing in as you do so.

3   Ensure your feet are about six inches off the ground and your shoulders about twelve inches off the ground and hold breathing naturally.

4   Now lift one leg higher than the other to about 12-18 inches, keeping your legs straight and interchange legs in an up and down motion. Use your arms for balance and concentration.

5   You can either pull your toes in towards you as you do this, or point them away from you in order to hit your muscles at varying angles.

6   Continue for as long as you can, rest and repeat for as many times as you are able.

The leg action is very similar to leg kicks when swimming backstroke.

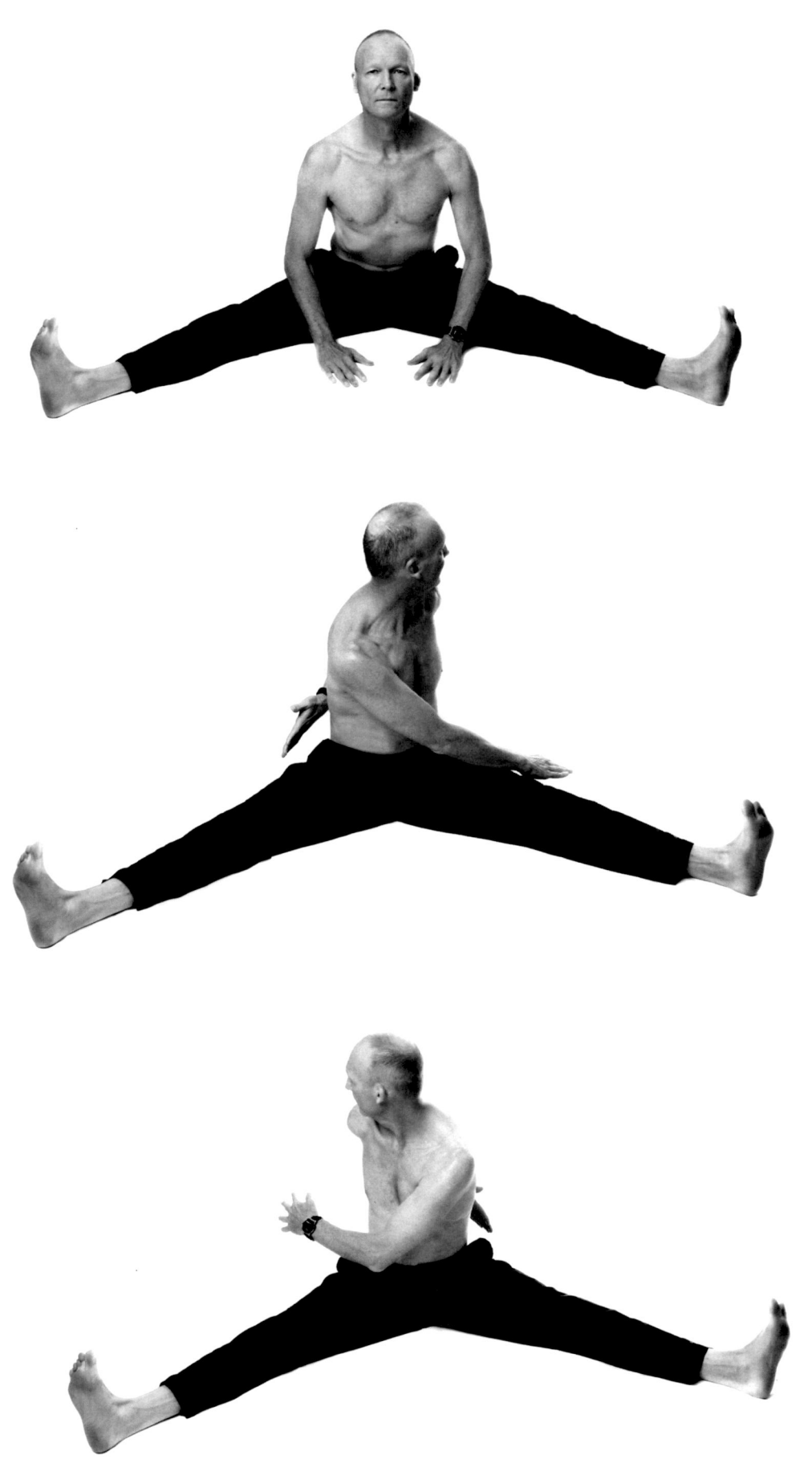

Fighting Fit Abs - Battle Proven Exercises

SEATED OPEN LEG TWISTS

This exercise will strengthen and loosen your obliques and destroy fat from your waist. It will also dramatically improve the strength in your upper body and back.

1   Sit on the ground with your legs open and the back of your legs in contact with the ground.

2   Breathe in and turn your upper body to the left as far as you can, keeping your arms bent and using the momentum to gently slap (massage) your kidneys with the inside of your hand.

3   Return to centre, exhale and repeat other side.

4   Carry out 15-50 repetitions.

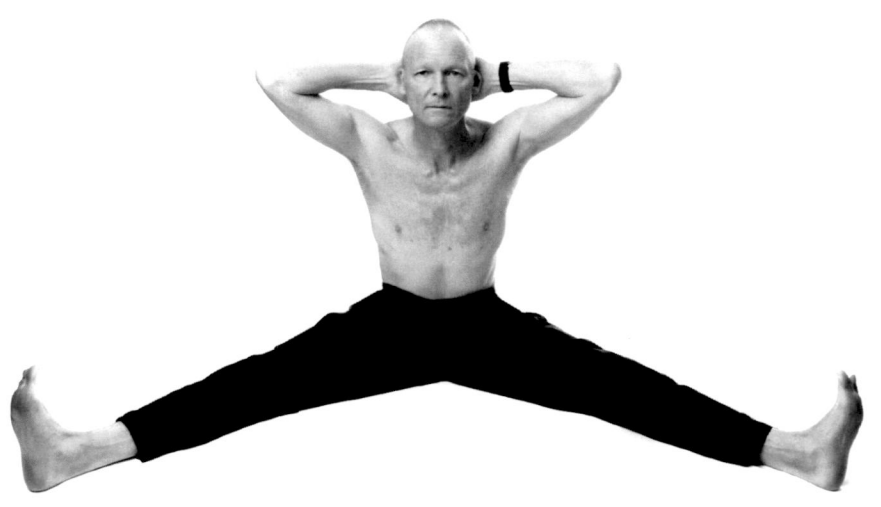

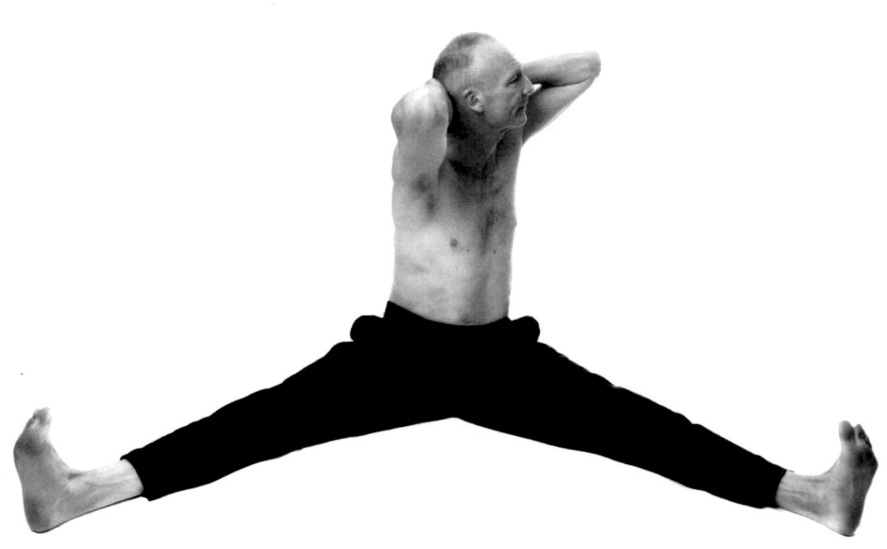

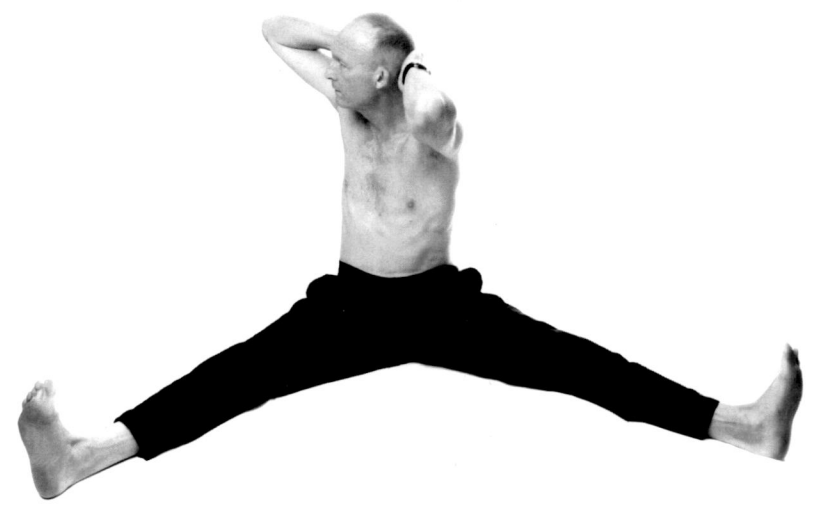

SEATED OPEN LEG TWISTS WITH HANDS BEHIND HEAD

This is similar to the previous exercise but with further emphasis on using your upper body and focusing in working your oblique's. It also helps to improve your posture and demolishes any flab from your waist.

1   Sit on the ground with your legs open and the back of your legs in contact with the ground and position your hands behind your head making sure that your elbows are pulled to the rear so that your spine remains straight.

2   Breathe in and turn your upper body to the left as far as you can ensuring that you do not use any momentum.

3   Return to the starting position and breathe out.

4   Repeat in the opposite direction.

5   Carry out 15-50 repetitions.

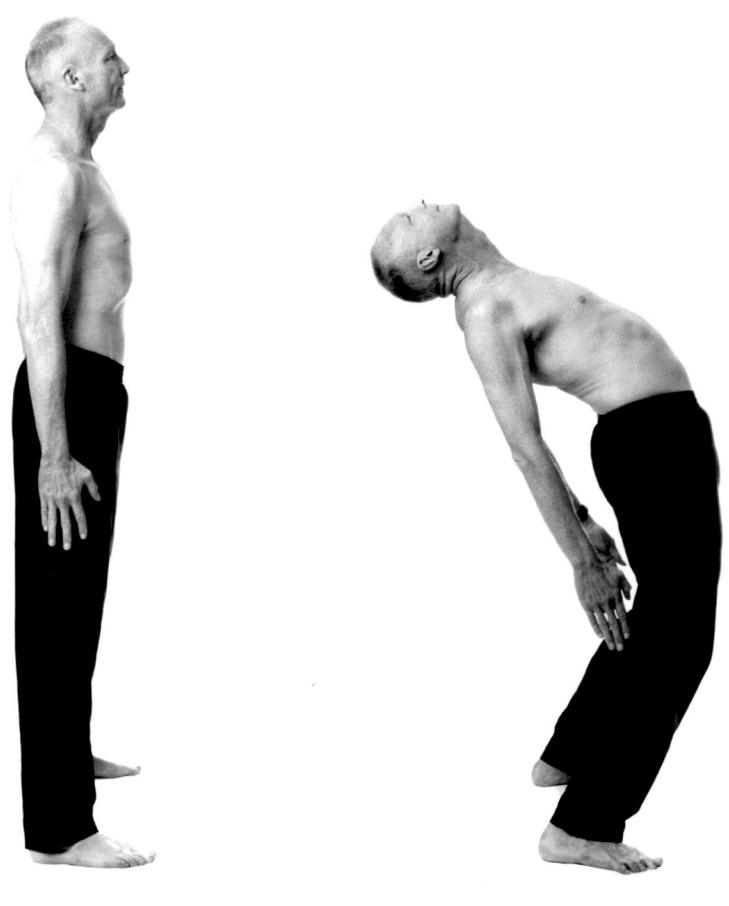

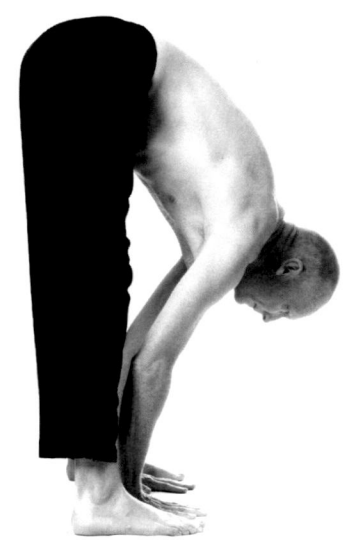

ISOMETRIC DOUBLE BACK BEND

Another exercise that strengthens and stretches your spine, lower back, abs, hamstrings and shoulders. It's a double whammy muscle builder and stomach flattener for you because it stretches your abs and spine in opposite directions and it contains tension techniques for further abdominal and body development.

1   Stand with your feet about shoulder width apart with arms hanging naturally.

2   Breathe in as deep as possible and lean back looking upwards as you do so.

3   Pause, hold and tense your abdominals and oblique's for 2-4 seconds.

4   Return to an upright position and then bend forward keeping your back and legs straight as you stretch with your hands to the ground.

5   Now squeeze your abs as hard as you can for 2-4 seconds.

6   Repeat this cycle 10-20 times.

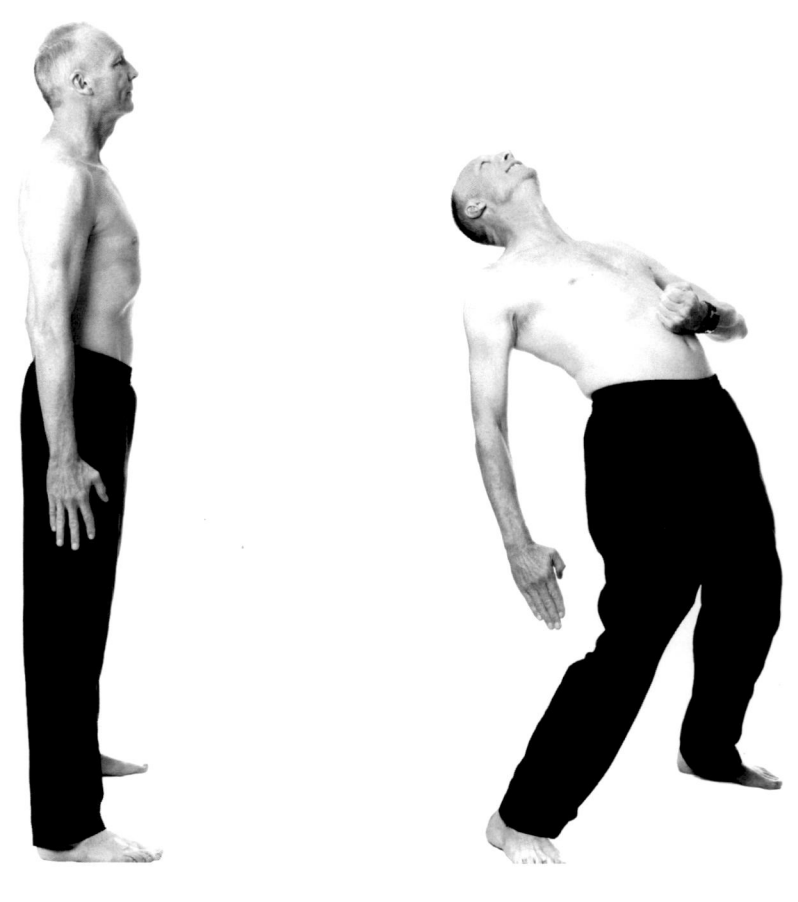

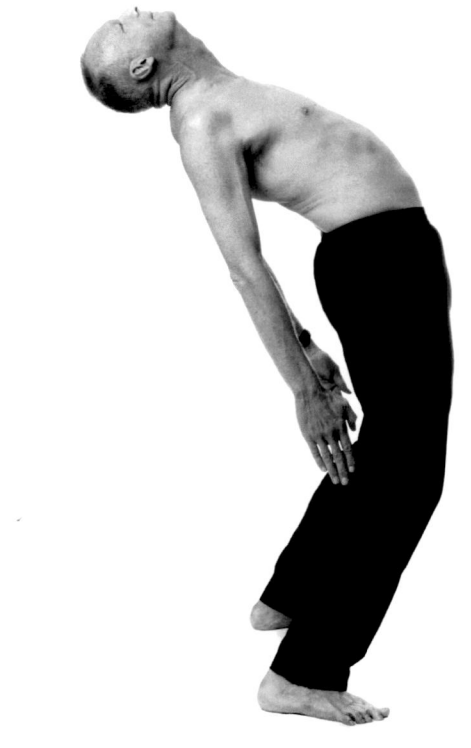

ISOMETRIC BACK BEND WITH IMPACT

Starts off the same as the previous exercise with the same benefits, but, you are going to strike yourself on your mid section – or you can ask someone else to do it for you! This is also a test to ensure that you are tensing your abs correctly; if you aren't, then you are in for a bit of a shock!

1   Stand with your feet about shoulder width apart with arms hanging naturally.

2   Breathe in as deep as possible and lean back looking upwards as you do so.

3   Pause, hold and tense your abdominals and oblique's hard and make impact to your abs with either the fleshy side of your fist (little finger end) or with the palm of your hand.

4   Do this 5-10 times each hand and then breathe out as you return to position 1 as above.

5   Repeat as often as you can.

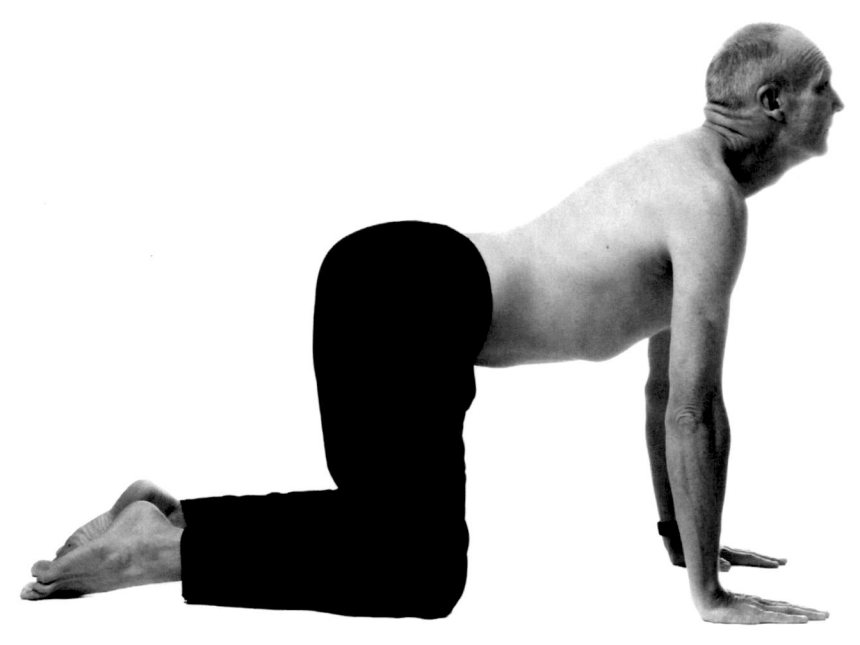

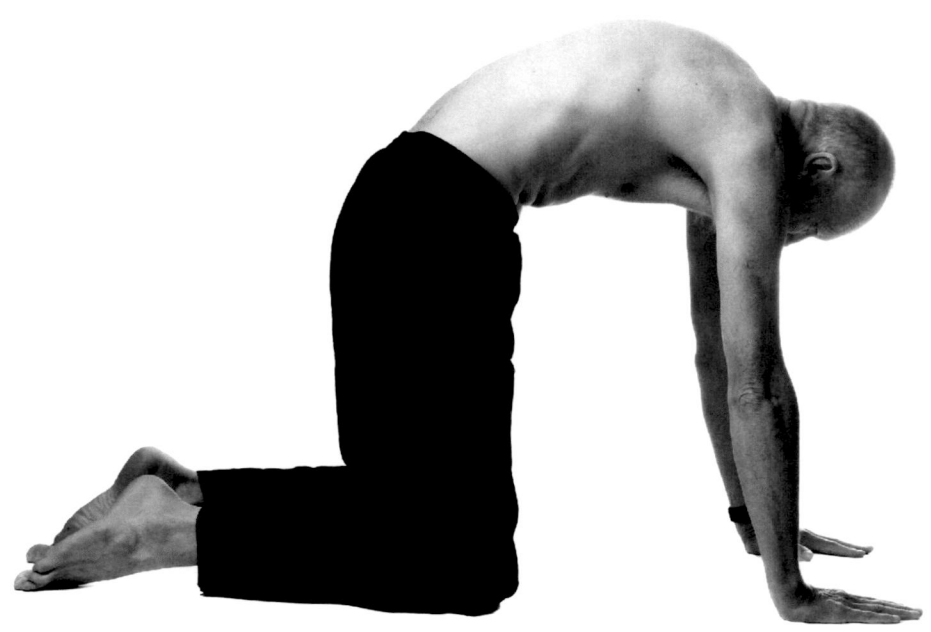

CAT STRETCH WITH ISOMETRIC SPINAL LIFT

This exercise targets your waistline and gives you a healthy spine, strong abs and a strong, loose lower back.

1   Start by kneeling on all fours with your body relaxed and your hips arched towards the ground so that your back is also arched inwards.

2   Expel all air out of your lungs.

3   Inhale deeply as you lift your diaphragm and stretch your spine upwards in a cat like motion.

4   Hold with strong tension for five seconds or longer.

5   Breathe out, relax and lower your spine.

6   Carry out 10-20 reps.

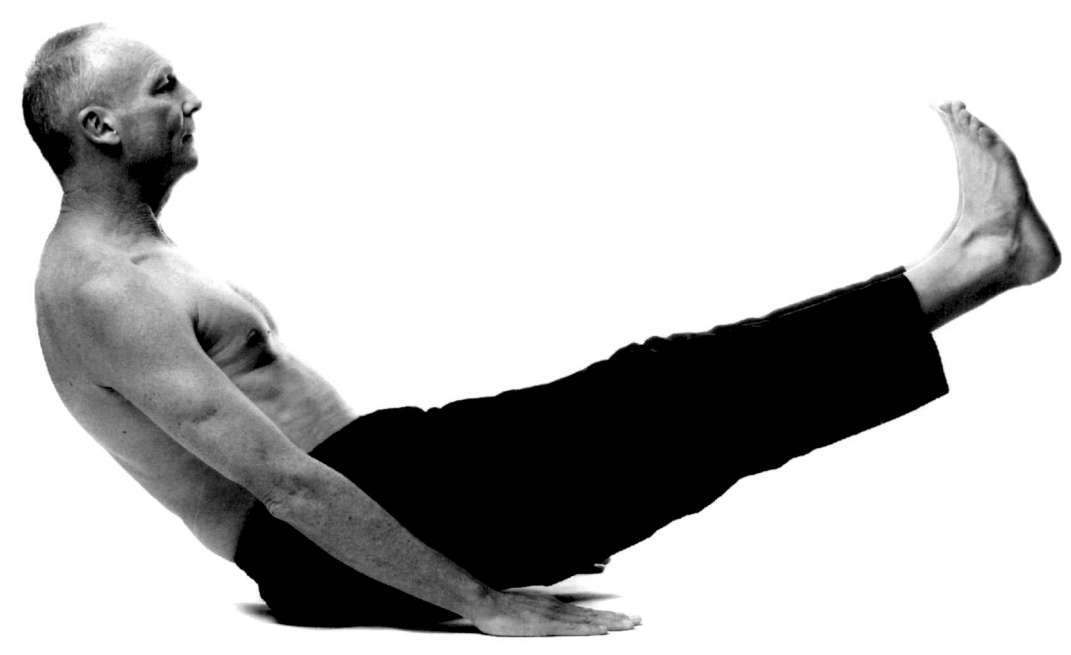

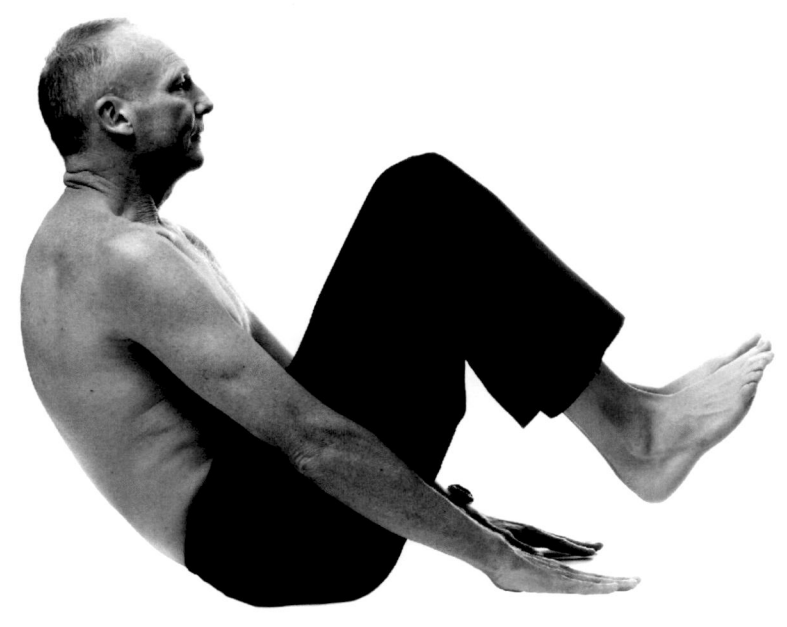

SHORT CURL UPS

**This curl up variation hits your upper and lower abs as well as your legs, lower back
and hip flexors. You need good co ordination for this.**

1   Get on your back with your legs straight and your arms at your sides.

2   Inhale and raise your legs and upper body off the ground and then pull your knees in towards your chest and hold.

3   Squeeze your abs in this position for 2-4 seconds.

4   Return to the start position, exhale and try and keep your legs and shoulders off the floor so that you have tension on your mid section throughout for maximum effect.

5   Repeat as many times as possible.

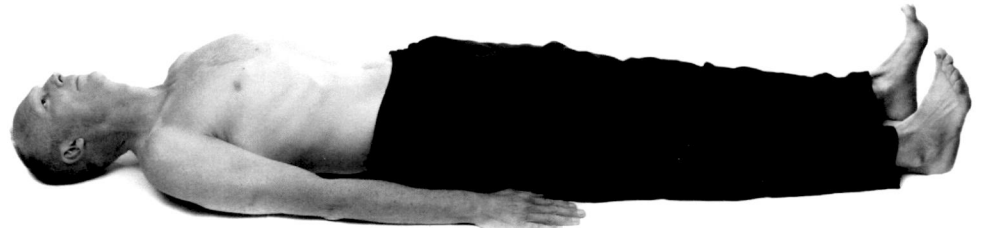

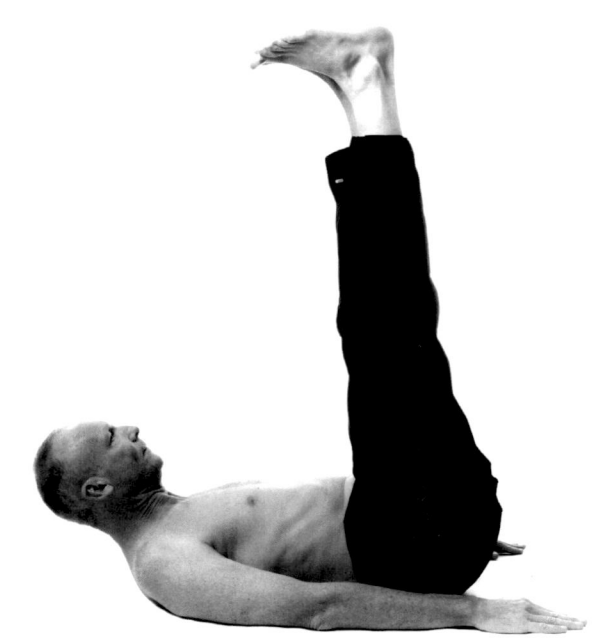

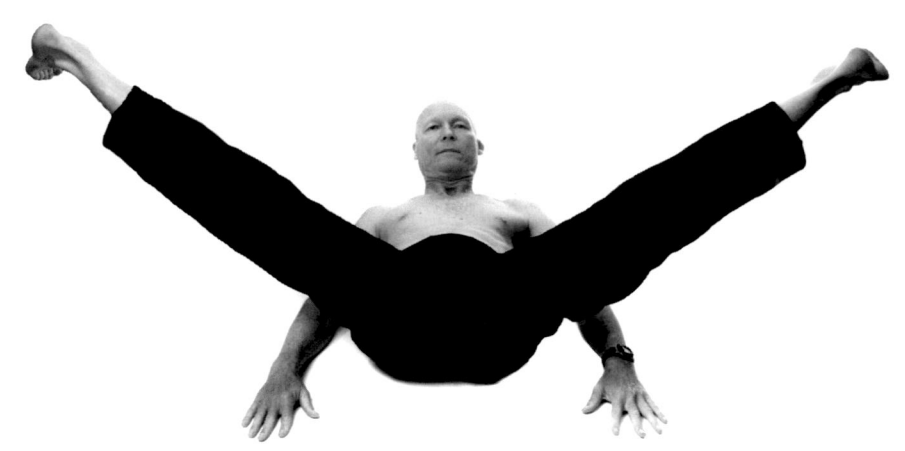

 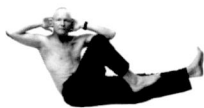

STRAIGHT LEG LIFTS

This one really hammers your abs – both upper and lower, and at the same time strengthening your lower back, neck and hip flexors; it hits them hard.

1   Once again, get down on your back and stretch out with your arms to your sides.

2   Look forward towards your feet and at the same time raise both legs straight with feet together to a vertical position.

3   Now tense your abs for a minimum of 2-5 seconds.

4   Open your legs keeping them straight and hold and tense as above.

5   Reverse the procedure and try not to rest your legs on the floor in between each exercise

6   Repeat for 10-50 reps.

7   Breathe out on the way up and out and then breathe in on the way down.

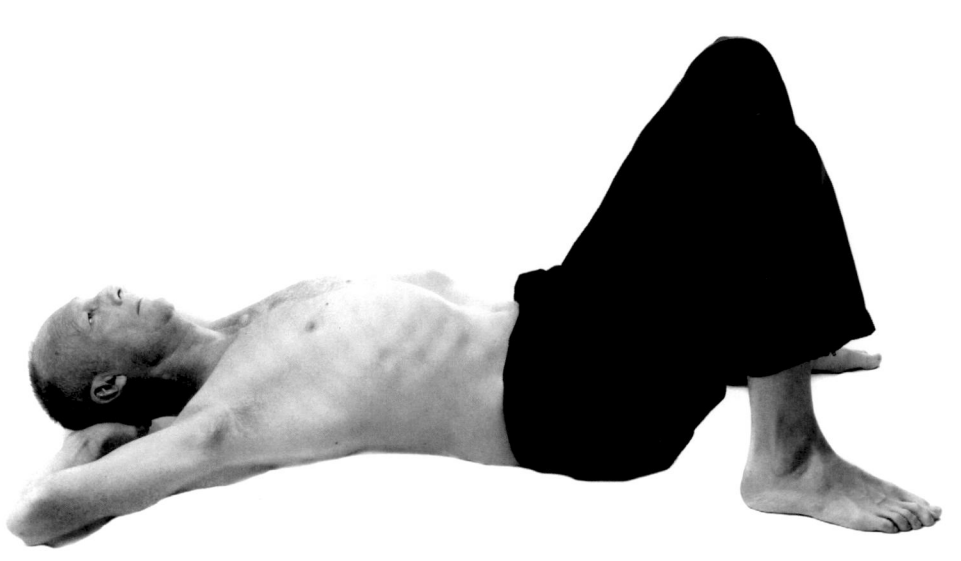

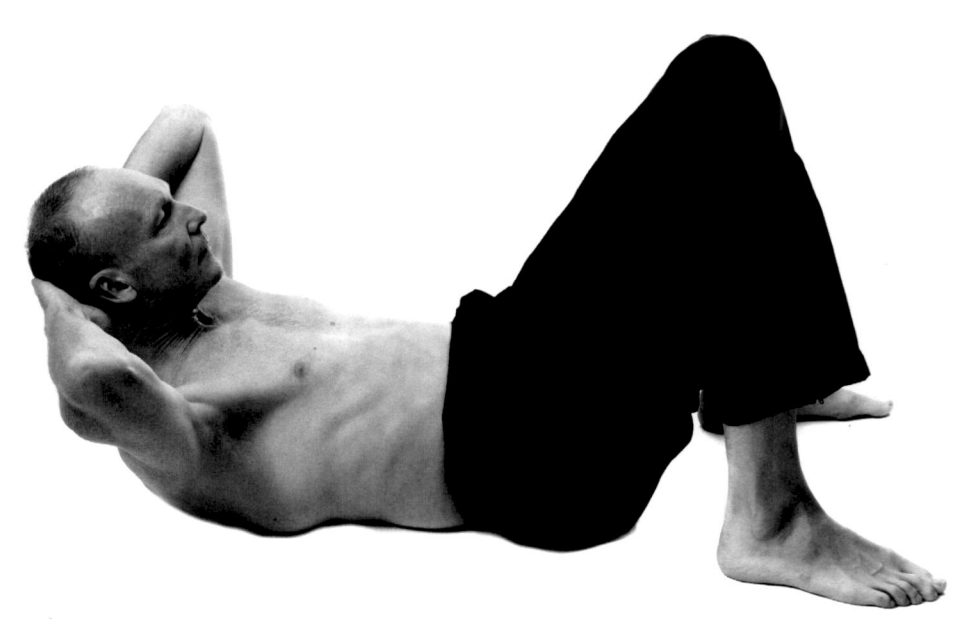

Fighting Fit Abs - Battle Proven Exercises

SHORT CURL UPS

Another 'top gun' abdominal exercise strength builder that blasts off stubborn belly flab.

1   Lie on your back with your legs bent and your feet drawn in as close as you are able to your buttocks.

2   Place your hands behind your head with fingers touching and elbows pulled back.

3   Exhale and roll your shoulders up off the floor a few inches only, making sure that your lower back stays on the ground.

4   Hold and tense for 2-4 seconds.

5   Lower your shoulders slowly and repeat without using momentum to bounce off the ground.

6   Do as many repetitions as you can.

Don't cheat as you are only cheating yourself.

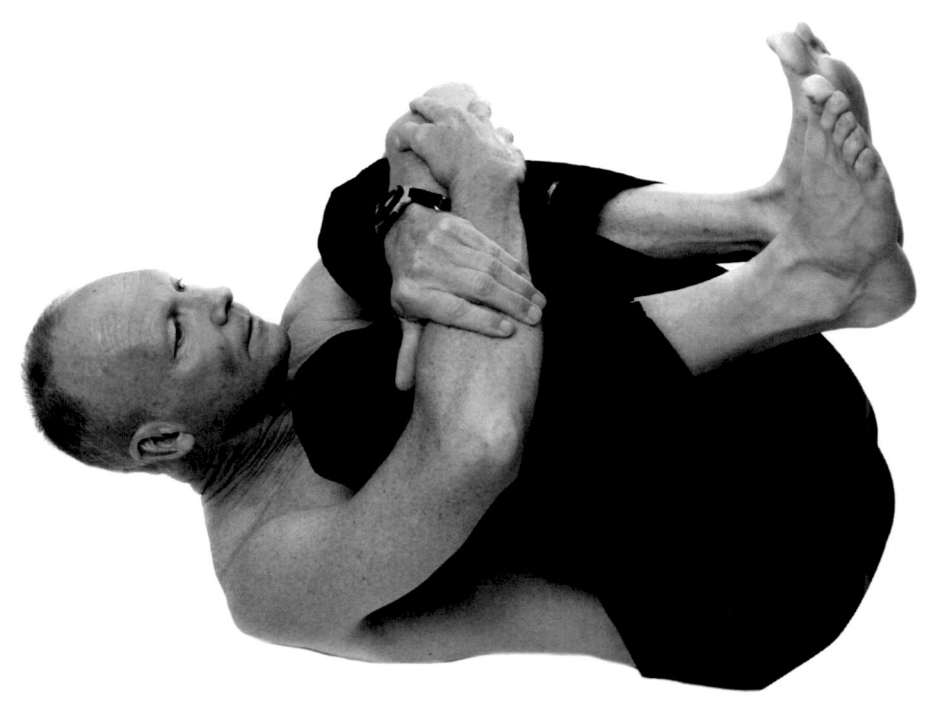

GRAB KNEES WITH TENSION

Ultimately, builds your abs, arms, shoulders and back... fast.

1 Adopt a position on your back, relax, breathe and visualise.

2 Lift your legs bent as far as you can towards your chest.

3 Reach out with your arms and grab your knees, pulling them into your chest as hard as you can.

4 Interlock your forearms and squeeze your abs, arms and shoulders hard. Hold for 5-10 seconds.

5 Repeat this whole drill as many times as you are able.

6 Exhale up and inhale down.

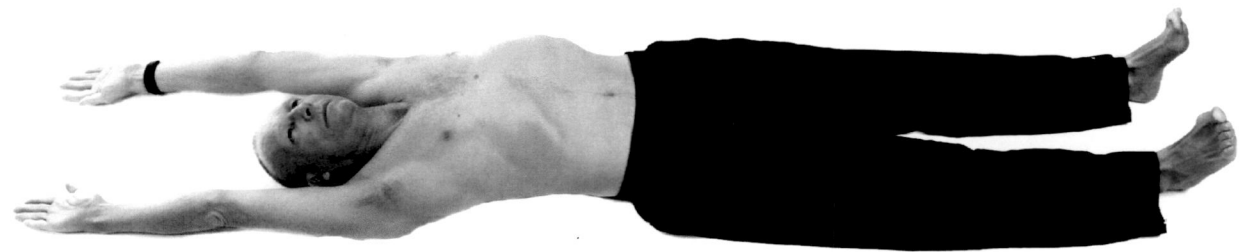

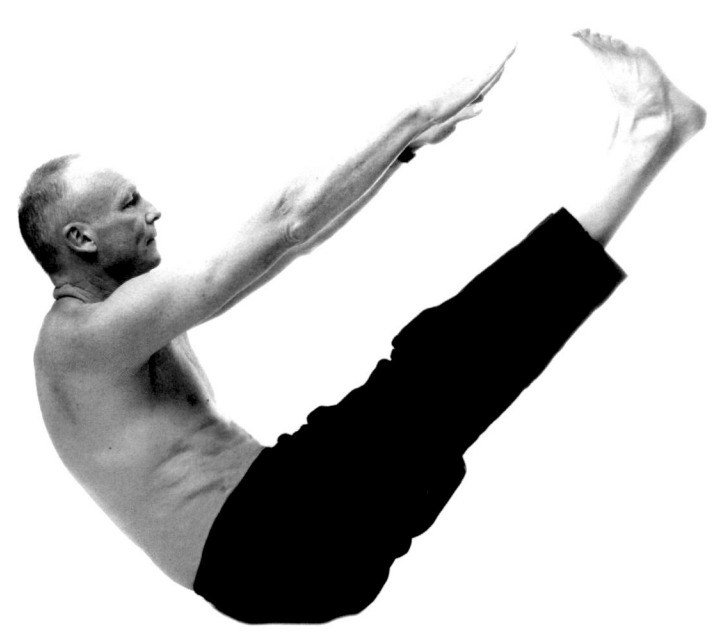

ISOMETRIC V-UP

This one really fires up your upper and lower abs – you really will feel as though they are on fire.

Exercises like this and other stuff that life tends to chuck at you, makes you mentally and physically tough, but only if you do what you have to do with confidence and commitment.

Challenge yourself to do what it takes to be a winner in your life.

1   Lie down on your back with your arms extended above your head and your legs straight.

2   Inhale at the same time as you simultaneously lift your legs and arms upwards and towards each other above your mid section.

3   Once you are in the highest balanced position you can get into, hold and squeeze your abs and breathe deeply.

4   Hold and squeeze for a minimum of 10-30 seconds and enjoy the 'fire' in your abs.

5   Just do 1-2 reps.

VERY IMPORTANT:

Go to my website at **www.MartinDayFitness.com** and provide me with your name and e-mail address so that I can send you a FREE fitness, health, motivation and training tip EVERY week. I promise to keep you positive, determined, informed and inspired. You won't believe how great they are until you get them so don't lose out. If you are serious about the "new you" that is, so don't delay, do it today.

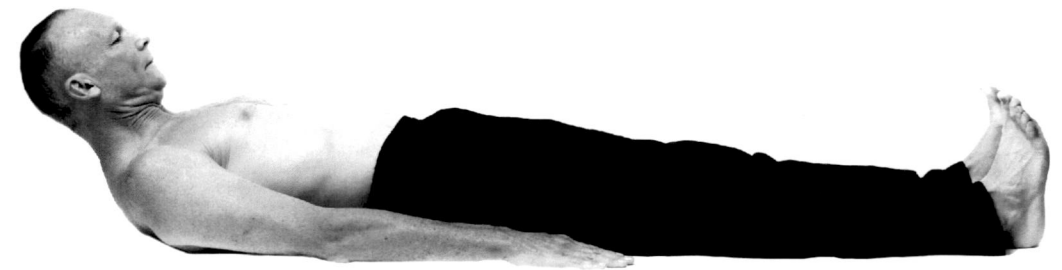

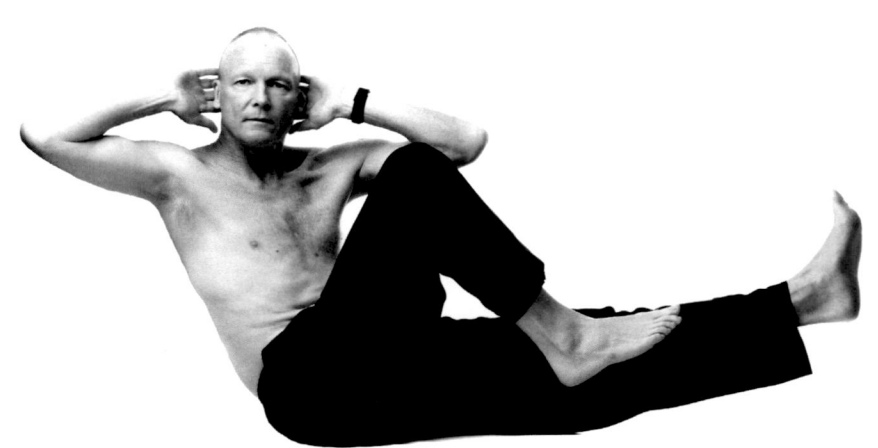

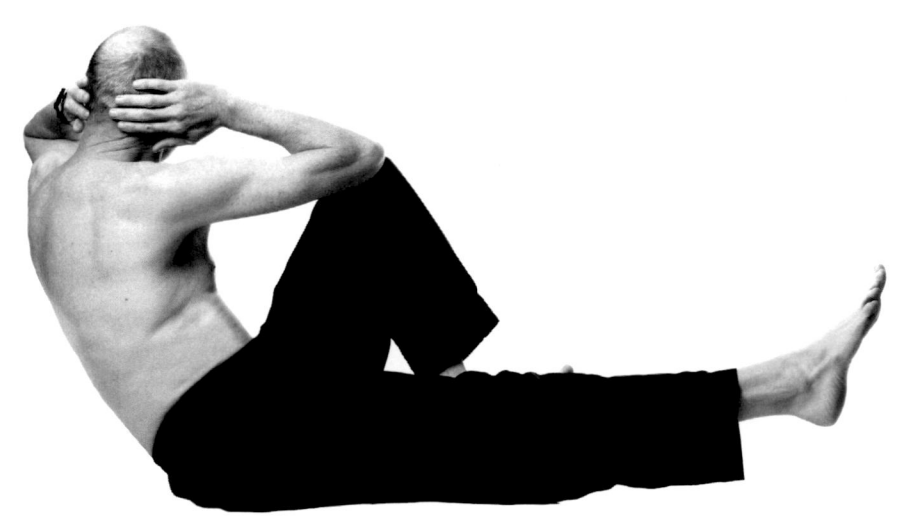

Fighting Fit Abs - Battle Proven Exercises

BENT LEG ALTERNATING CURL UPS

Once again you need co ordination to do this exercise and once again, it's a very effective upper and lower abs 'hitter.'

1   Get onto your back and stretch out with your arms to your sides.

2   Place your hands behind your head and exhale whilst lifting both legs a few inches off the ground.

3   As you curl up, drive your right leg in towards your chest with your left leg off the ground.

4   At the same time twist your left elbow towards your right knee as far as you can.

5   Tense your abs in this position before exhaling and returning to the starting position.

6   Repeat with your left leg and right elbow.

7   Do as many reps as you can.

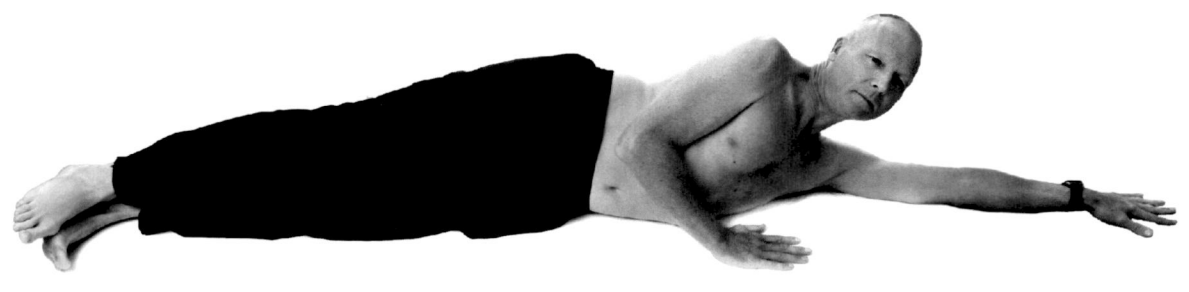

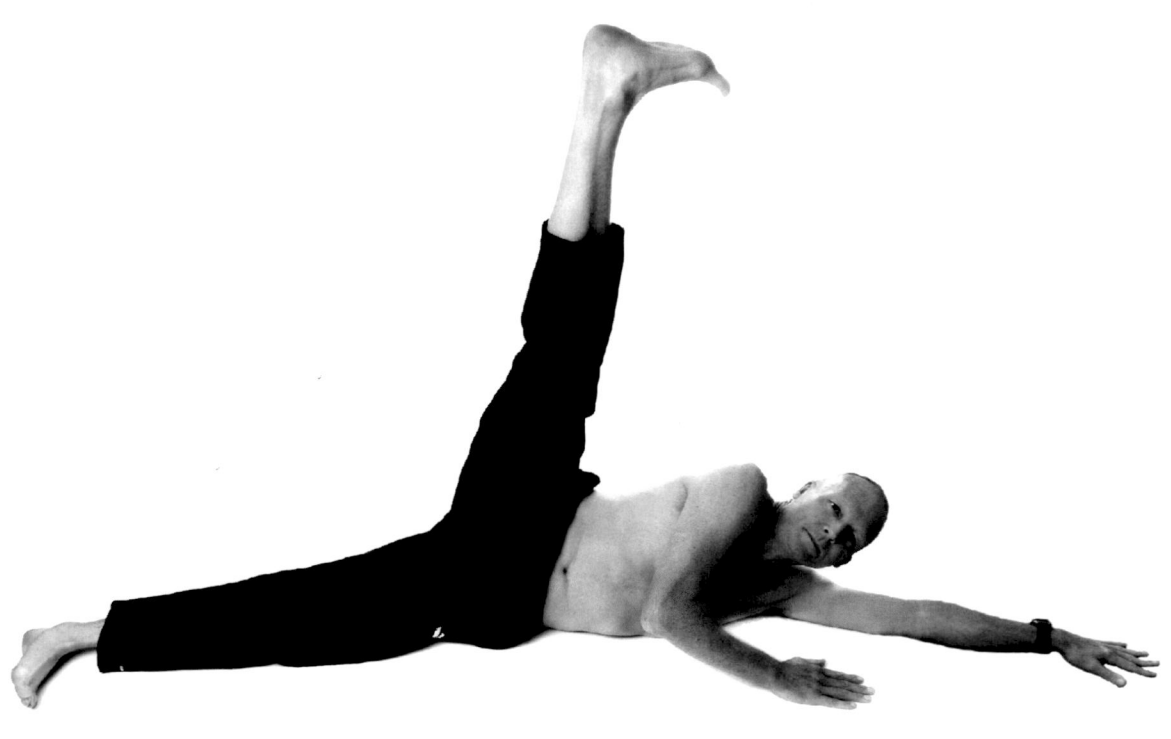

Fighting Fit Abs - Battle Proven Exercises

SIDE LEG LIFTS

More co-ordination and balance needed from you for this exercise which will dynamite your abs, oblique's, legs and hip flexors.

1   Lie on your side with legs straight and together with your left am extended and in line with your body. Use your other arm to keep your balance in front of your chest.

2   Exhale and lift your straight right leg as high as you can and in line towards your extended arm.

3   Hold this position and tense your upper and lower abs and oblique's as hard as you can for 2-5 seconds.

4   Inhale as you slowly lower your right leg and repeat a minimum of 5-10 times.

5   Change sides and repeat.

Note: If you want to target and build other muscles – then turn your raised foot inwards with your big toe pointed at the ground.

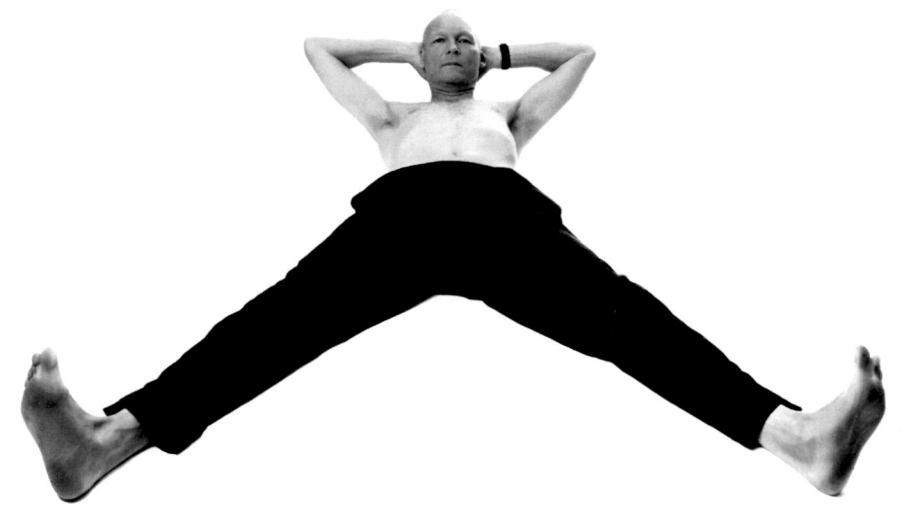

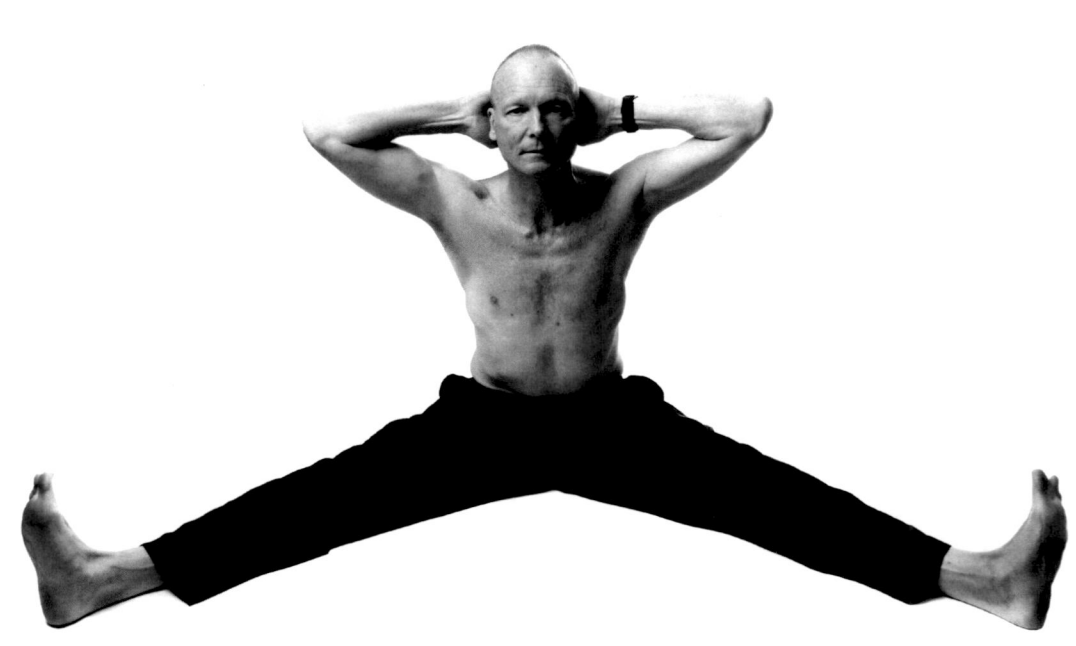

WIDE LEG CURL UPS

Another very demanding but beneficial exercise that promotes flexibility in your hips as well as building your abdominal muscles.

1   Lie on you back with your legs wide apart and your hands behind your head.

2   Try not to use your arms to curl up and ensure that your legs stay on the ground – use your abs only.

3   Curl your upper body all the way up so that it is at a right angle to your legs.

4   Slowly lower yourself back to the starting position ensuring that you use your stomach muscles to control this movement.

5   Repeat as many times as possible.

6   Breathe out up and breathe in down.

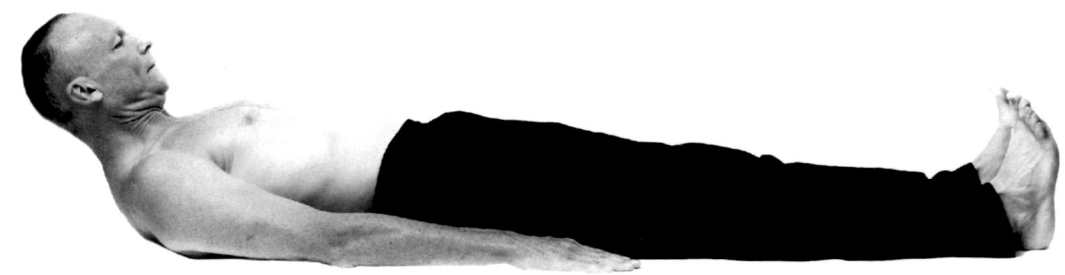

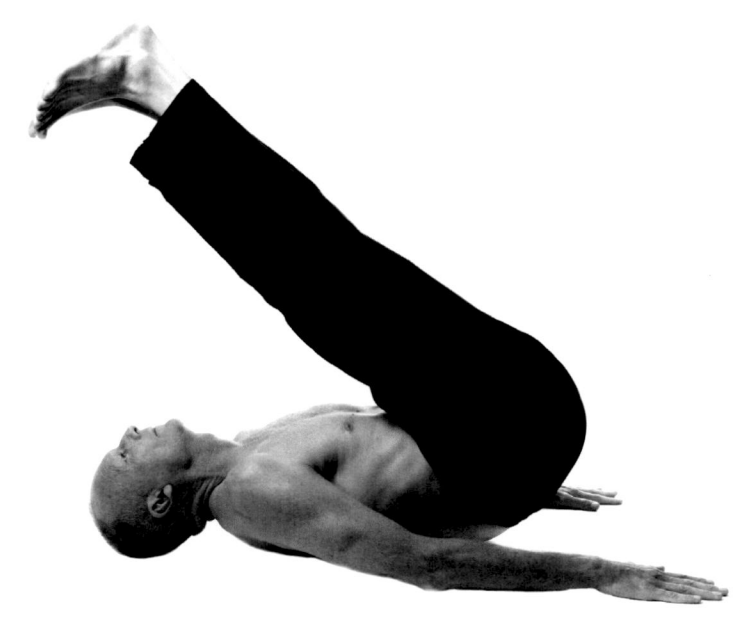

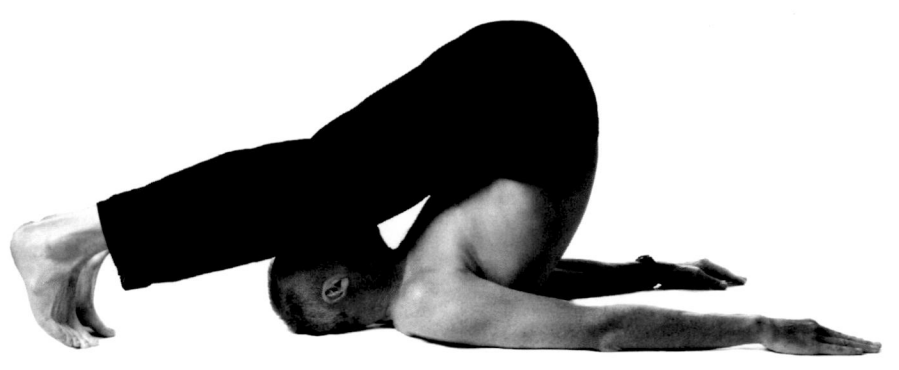

Fighting Fit Abs - Battle Proven Exercises

LEG LIFTS BEHIND HEAD

I learned this exercise from a SBS (Special Boat Squadron) officer and it's a great back, legs, neck and abs strengthener. You will also make landmark gains in your hamstring and lower back flexibility.

1   Adopt a position on your back with legs straight and your arms to your sides.

2   Lift both of your legs together and straight as high as you can and back towards your head.

3   Hold and tense your abs for about 2-5 seconds.

4   Continue to drive your legs straight towards and above your head, hold and tense as above.

5   Return to start position and repeat.

6   Breathe deep as best you can.

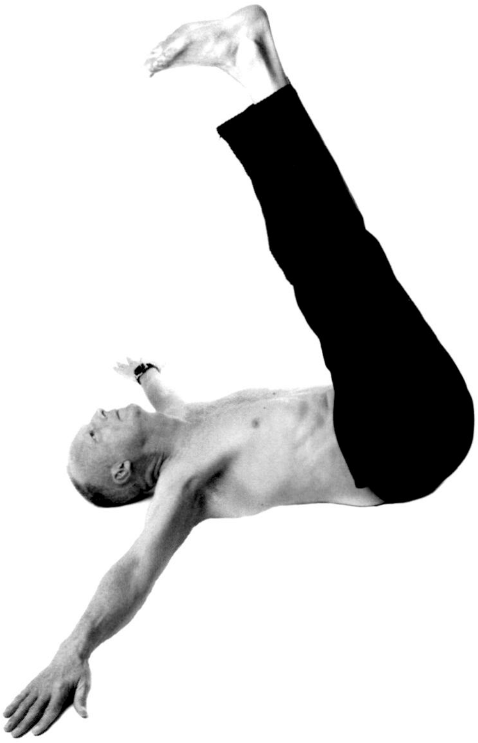

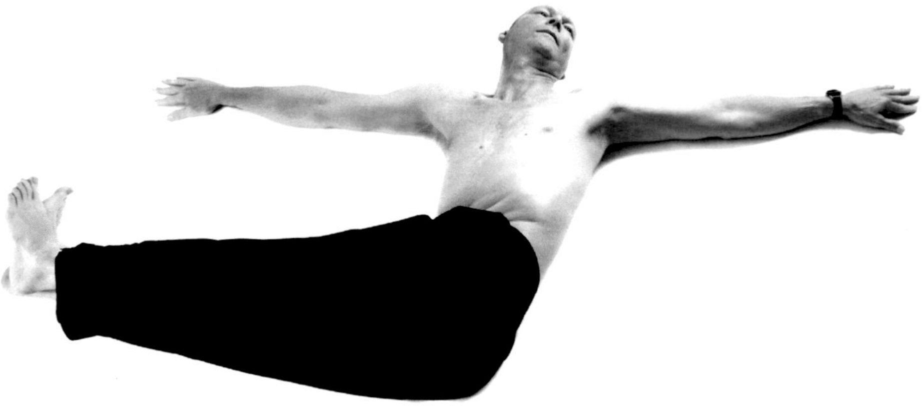

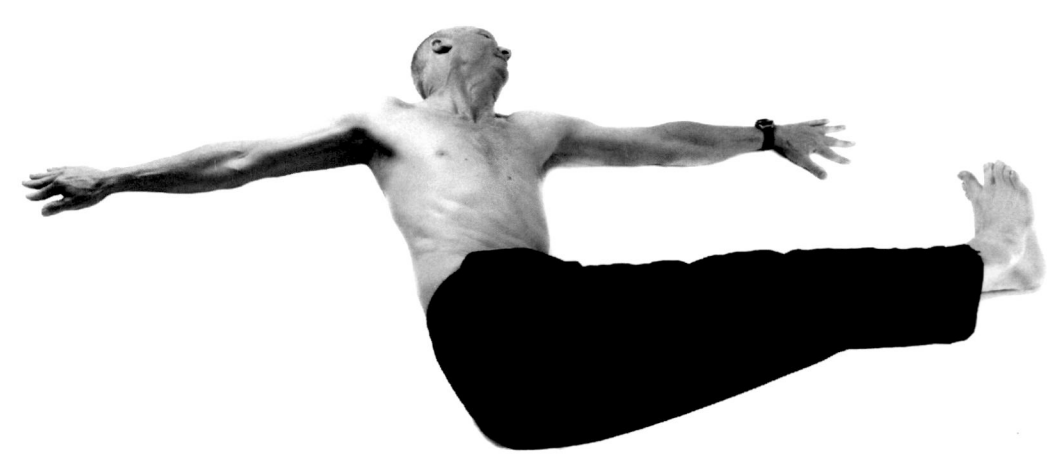

Fighting Fit Abs - Battle Proven Exercises

ANGULAR ROTATIONS

This is a formidable abs builder that also guarantees to strengthen your legs, sides and hip flexors. Make sure that you use your hands for balance and be prepared for super gains in your flexibility.

1 Lie on your back with your arms to your sides.

2 Inhale and raise both legs up to a vertical position and then across to your right side.

3 Hold and tense your abs in this position.

4 Raise your legs to a vertical position again and then across to your left side.

5 Hold this position and tense.

6 Breathe naturally throughout as you do this exercise.

7 Carry out 10 repetitions in each direction.

Note: Do not rest your legs on the floor when you lift them to each side of you.

FREQUENTLY ASKED QUESTIONS

How will the Exercises help me?

All of the exercises shown in this book will strengthen all of your muscles including your spine and extremities and of course your mid section and core. Your digestive system and internal organs will also benefit and each and every day you will notice physical and psychological gains.

Am I In Safe Physical Condition to do these Exercises?

The exercises are for everyone who is healthy and at any age, including 50s, 60s and older. If in doubt about your health, especially if you have any joint problems speak to your physician first.

What do I Wear (Order of Dress) and do I need any Equipment?

Wear the most comfortable clothing that you have and don't load too much on unless you are training outside and there is snow on the ground. Dress in shorts, t-shirt, sweat top, socks and shoes or train barefoot inside as this will give you added strength in your feet and ankles.

No exercise equipment is needed apart from a towel, a bottle of water and maybe a mat for when you are exercising on your back, front or side.

How often should I do the exercises?

Do a little each day or every other day without being lazy. Broadly speaking though, you will need to spend about 15 to 20 minutes per day on the Fighting Fit exercises featured in this book. When you start you may not be able to do 15 to 20 minutes. Do what you can. Begin slowly and then progress to higher levels of strength, fitness and flexibility.

"Perfection is not an essential ingredient for success"

Vitally Important Exercises

These are the HIT LIST. You may not be able to do them very well at first; don't worry, and don't let this stop you. When I first began training with them, my technique was not very good but I have persevered and I am still improving. Don't hang around waiting for your technique to be ideal or you will be waiting for a long time. The most important thing is that you START your training.

Dear Friend

I know the 2008 Olympics have finished but I just had to fire off what really stood out to me during that time.

It's about Michael Phelps - one of history's now very legendary swimmers and how he can stay lean, fit and muscular; especially around his mid section even though he eats ten thousand calories a day worth of food and drink... Sounds unbelievable doesn't it?

The truth is - that's what he gets through during the day.

I pulled this info out of the paper – this is what he eats for breakfast:
'three fried egg sandwiches, with cheese, tomatoes, lettuce, fried onions and mayonnaise, as well as three chocolate chip pancakes; a five-egg omelette; three sugar-coated slices of french toast, a bowl of cereal and two cups of coffee.'

So, the big question is....Why doesn't he have fat hanging everywhere by eating this amount of calorie loaded food? The answer is really straightforward and it isn't rocket science... Here's the thing; he trains every day and goes really hard at it, which results in him burning off huge amounts of calories.

Phelps also has a fast metabolism that blasts the fat off his body 24/7, keeping his body lean and   athletic.

Can we do this?

Unfortunately, most of us won't be able to torch off that amount of calories, but, remember - the more you work out using high energy techniques -in other words, blast your training hard and get a major sweat on, then the less you have to worry about how much you eat.

This is the way to burn calories - exercise HARD during workouts and get your metabolism cranked up and working. So don't feel guilty about having a splurge now and again!

If you have a really active metabolism and can eat anything you want without gaining an ounce - then there is nothing more for me to say.....

But, if you've been plagued with being out of shape. If you've got a bit of a belly hanging and you want to eat like 'Mr and Mrs Slim' living down the road and not have to be on a starvation diet and watch every single thing you eat, then you need to train hard with my Fighting Fit training system:

www.MartinDayFitness.com

This is the answer to the new you. It really works!

Be the best!

Martin Day

Bodybuilding Muscles

In my experience, most bodybuilders do not have conditioned and functional muscles like an athlete. They are muscle bound and find it difficult to move fast and they lack agility. Fighting Fit exercises are designed for you to get workable fitness. With that it means strength, agility, stamina and flexibility. I have taught bodybuilders and weight lifters in my martial arts sessions and they suffer lack of endurance and, believe it or not, they are the first to get injured and usually the first to "wimp out" of training. So what does this tell you? Train with the bodyweight exercises contained in Fighting Fit, if you want functional fitness. They will look after you for life.

How Many Repetitions do I do and for How Long?

Do as many as you can and for as long as you can but don't go over the top when you first start as you will be sore for a few days. I have indicated the minimum number of repetitions or a time stipulation for the exercises; do the best you can and don't waver. What is the maximum then? Well, there is no maximum as the human mind and body is capable of great things. Set yourself a target with the HIT LIST and go to it. The feeling of achievement is like no other when you exceed what you couldn't previously do.

Why is drinking lots of water so important?

Most of your body is made up of water and we lose vast quantities of it every day, especially when we are doing physical exercise. It therefore makes sense that we have to replace it otherwise we're in trouble. You should be drinking on average eight glasses a day, more when you are training.

Another thing that I have learned over the years is to sip water through the day and when you eat. Don't fall into the trap of drinking gallons of the stuff before, during and after meals as you will feel heavy and bloated. Test it out and you will see what I mean.

How can I lose weight faster?

If I were you I would get my other book Secrets of Fighting Fit Exposed – Battle Proven Conditioning Exercises for Strength, Fitness and Flexibility. It contains very intensive workout routines and dynamic exercises that will work wonders for you. I also explain interval and skipping rope training in my book but my advice is if you mix say, a 200 metre sprint with 20 sit ups and press ups, then sprint 100 metres and do 20 squat thrusts and astride jumps then you will be where you want to be in no time. Just focus and get rid of all outside thoughts and distractions and concentrate on what you want to achieve.

When Do I Stop Training?

You don't! I train every day and it is part of my daily routine, just like getting dressed in the morning and brushing my teeth. Every athlete and go getter will tell you that they achieve success because they are in a routine. Daily exercise should be a lifelong commitment and something to enjoy and not something to try and get away from.

I Don't Like Exercise But Can I Still Benefit From Your Natural Eating Plan Only?

Of course – getting the right nutrition is very important. Just remember that the way to a long healthy life and the secret to fat loss is to EXERCISE and EAT SENSIBLY and to stretch. The other crucial factor is to be determined and have a positive mind. I hope you change your mind and start exercising.

Why Do People Get Fatter as They Get Older?

Simply because they become inactive using age, family and work commitments as an excuse not to do anything physical. The answer of course is to do something that activates the metabolism on a regular basis and to eat sensibly. I know seventy year olds that are in fantastic shape and have a great lust for life because they train regularly. Have a look around you and you'll see what I mean.

I've been Invited To a Party with the Temptation of Lots of Food and Drink, What Do I Do?

Get along there, enjoy yourself and let your hair down. One evening of indulgence a week won't do you any harm. Actually, it's good that you splurge now and again as it keeps you positive and focused so don't feel guilty.

Why is a Pot or Beer Belly Dangerous to Health?

Men are at risk of getting a big fat gut and they then have a massive chance of getting heart disease, diabetes, gallstones and some types of cancer. This is now classed as the most dangerous form of obesity. Females tend to store fat around their buttocks and hips. The good news is that if an exercise program – like mine is followed, even losing a few kilos of fat could save your life.

Don't waste time

The worse thing that you can do is to flake out in front of the tele in the evening. Nothing has ever been gained from playing computer games, watching DVDs or surfing the net. Instead, take advantage of the opportunity to work off your dinner by doing some exercises. It also de stresses you and clears your mind.

A SNEAK PEEK AT OTHER MARTIN DAY PRODUCTS

SECRETS OF FIGHTING FIT EXPOSED 3

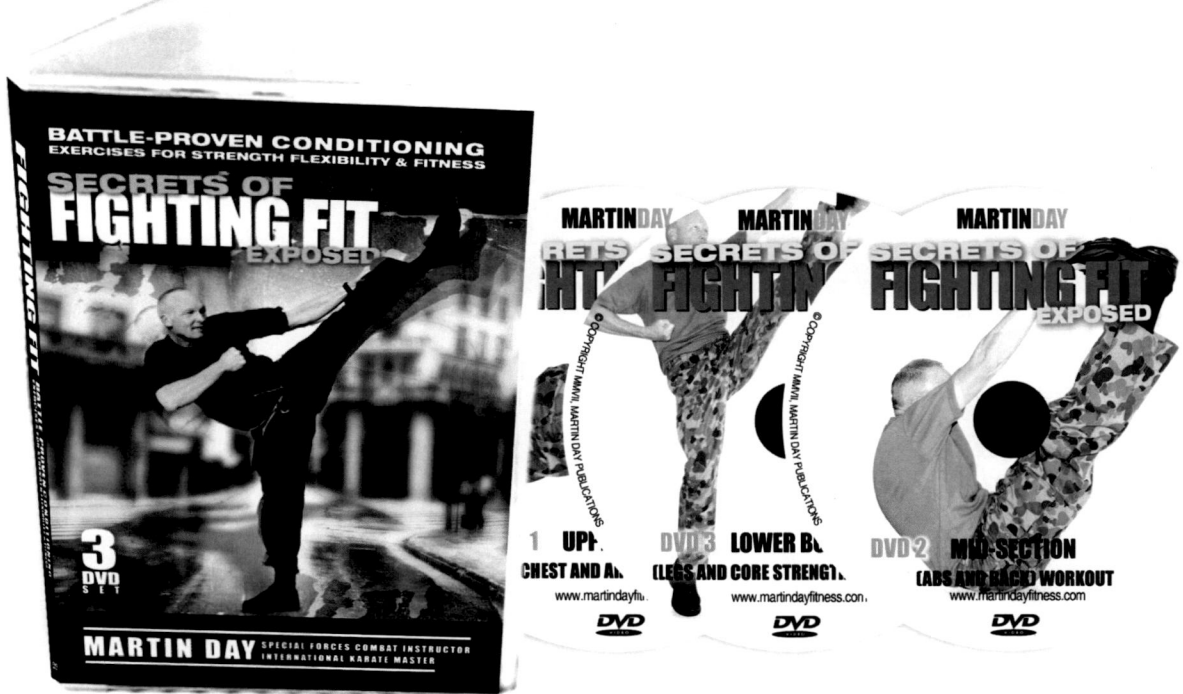

Amazing Results...

These 3 Powerful DVD's take you through the exercises contained within the 160 page book **Secrets of Fighting Fit Exposed: Battle Proven Conditioning Exercises For Strength Flexibility & Fitness**. PLUS extra exercises and training tips for even faster results.

Maximum results in the shortest possible time!

"I feel like a NEW PERSON"   **- Jane Ingham**

"'I lost 8 kg in 4 weeks, was motivated to quit smoking and to live a healthier life. As such I highly recommend these DVDs to anyone who is serious about getting results fast!"   **- Colin Arthur**

These powerful DVDs also show the BATTLE GROUP – the 3 exercises that will change your life – along with supremely effective bodyweight exercises and workouts that will get you seeing and feeling the results straight away.

Make no mistake these DVDs will get you in awesome shape FAST!

YOU CAN CONTACT US IN THE FOLLOWING WAYS:

Martin Day Publications
Secure On-Line Ordering at
www.MartinDayFitness.com

Snail Mail for ALL Correspondence and Orders:
Martin Day Publications
Suite 8, Noosa Boardroom
28 Eenie Creek Rd
Noosaville Queensland 4566, Australia

Call 24 hrs:

Within Australia
Tel: 1300 851 401
Fax: 07 5430 6677

International:
Phone: + 61 7 5430 6662
Fax: + 61 7 5430 6677

KILLER POWER KICKS AND PUNCHES

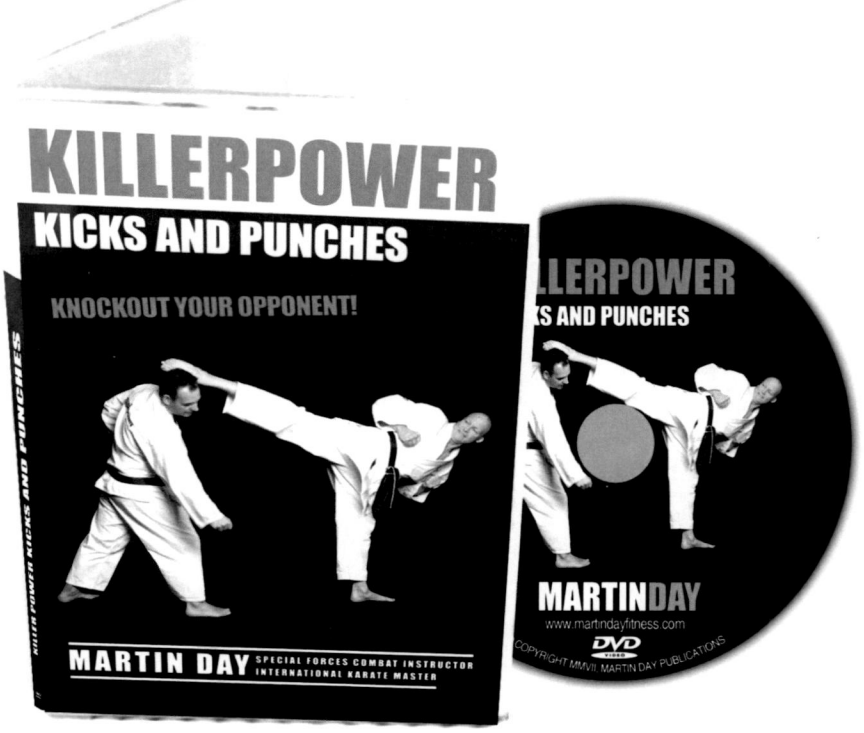

Ultra-Effective Tournament Techniques…

Bone-Crushing Tournament Winning techniques that will destroy your competitors (or an attacker on the street). This DVD highlights 62 never before revealed combinations that have been used to win International competitions.

Follow step-by-step as each combination is revealed in dynamic non-stop action by Shihan (Master) Martin Day 5th Dan Black Belt.

"I used these techniques to win major International titles, they are the best out there and they just demolish the opposition!"

- Patricia Fast 4th Dan – International Black Belt Kumite Champion

"You owe it to yourself to gain a huge advantage in your training – if you are serious that is…. that's why I use the techniques shown – they work brilliantly, just do it!"

- David Rowe 3rd Kyu – National All Styles Championships 1st Place

YOU CAN CONTACT US IN THE FOLLOWING WAYS:

Martin Day Publications
Secure On-Line Ordering at
www.MartinDayFitness.com

Snail Mail for ALL Correspondence and Orders:
Martin Day Publications
Suite 8, Noosa Boardroom
28 Eenie Creek Rd
Noosaville Queensland 4566, Australia

Call 24 hrs:

Within Australia
Tel: 1300 851 401
Fax: 07 5430 6677

International:
Phone: + 61 7 5430 6662
Fax: + 61 7 5430 6677

UNCENSORED ELITE UNARMED COMBAT 3

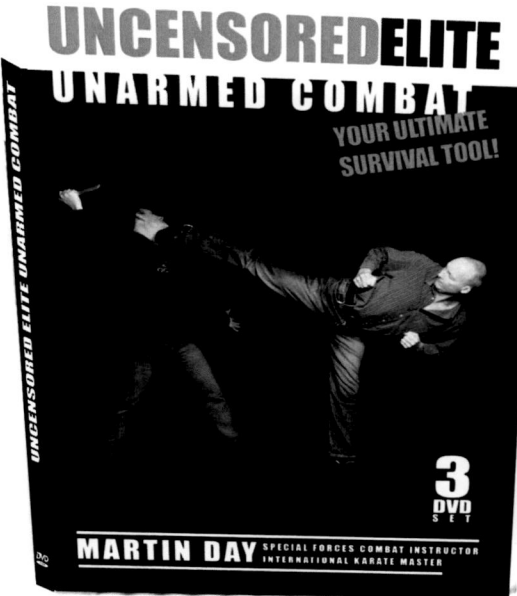
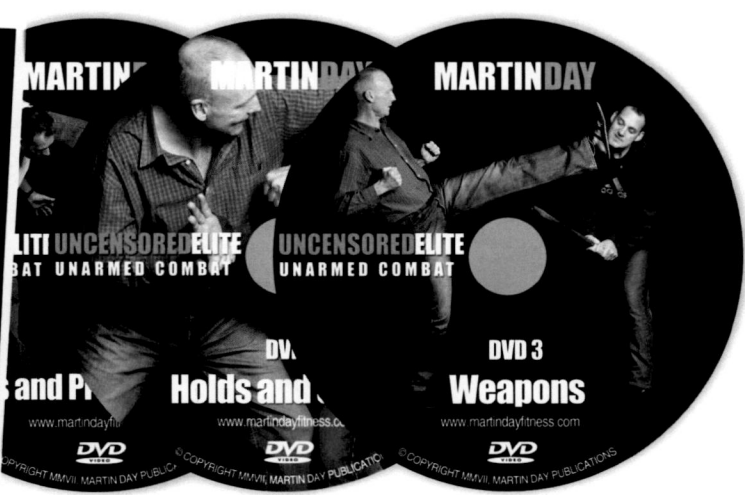

Easily Destroy Your Attackers...

Discover 106 life preserving unarmed combat techniques that YOU can use to ***TAKE OUT*** any scumbags

to protect yourself, your family and your friends.

Nothing else on the market gets close to what's revealed in this DVD set!

| **DVD 1** | **DVD 2** | **DVD 3** |
| **Grabs & Pressure Points** | **Holds & Strikes** | **Weapons** |

"I was attacked by two yobs using weapons and I used the techniques shown in these DVDs to save myself from serious injury...they are the real deal!"
- M. Robinson

"Three muggers demanded my wallet and my mobile phone as I left a train station in broad daylight. I had the ability, confidence and posture through learning the techniques in this DVD to defend myself; I am forever thankful"
- C. Coenen

"I can't thank Martin enough, his training is light years ahead of anything else out there and he has given me shed loads of confidence."
- P. Fast

YOU CAN CONTACT US IN THE FOLLOWING WAYS:

Martin Day Publications
Secure On-Line Ordering at
www.MartinDayFitness.com

Snail Mail for ALL Correspondence and Orders:
Martin Day Publications
Suite 8, Noosa Boardroom
28 Eenie Creek Rd
Noosaville Queensland 4566, Australia

Call 24 hrs:

Within Australia
Tel: 1300 851 401
Fax: 07 5430 6677

International:
Phone: + 61 7 5430 6662
Fax: + 61 7 5430 6677

ULTIMATE FIGHTING FIT FLEXIBILITY TECHNIQUES

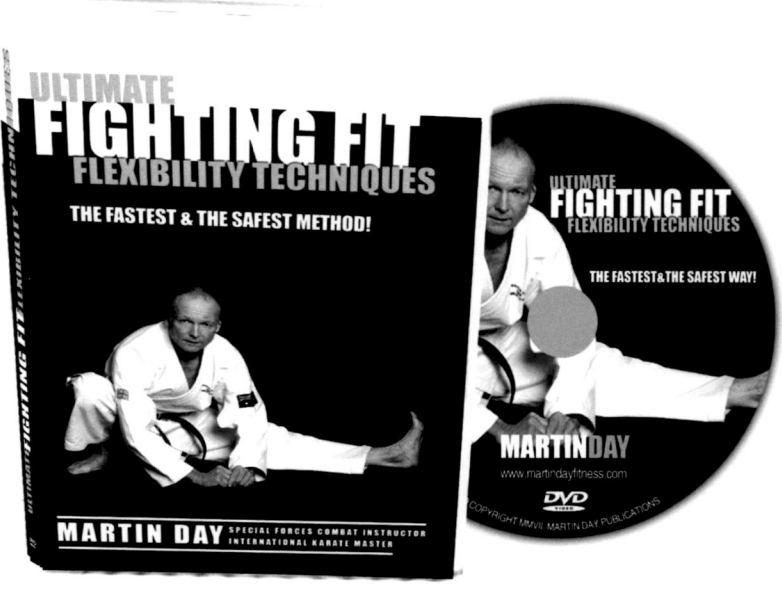

Learn how to gain awesome, animal-like flexibility, loosen up those stiff joints and release all that junk in your muscles, restoring them back to their youthful and healthy state.

In Only A Few Minutes A Day!

"I have found the techniques so effective that I've made the exercises the lynchpin of both my personal and my martial arts club training. Martin Day doesn't just teach exercises, Fighting Fit Conditioning is a philosophy of physical culture that stands on its own and will help ANYONE with the guts to give it a real go!"

— M Boardman

"Wow, I can't believe it, my flexibility has more than trebled after only two sessions! As a 48 year old who has never been flexible this is a revelation – and I am so much stronger. I wake up with more energy and I am enjoying life even more, if I can do it anyone can!"

— L Capinnell

Minutes after doing these workouts, you're going to have greater flexibility and power in your whole body that you never thought possible. You will also have real fire in your belly, and be full of get up and go enthusiasm that had inexplicably ebbed out of you, without you even realising it.

YOU CAN CONTACT US IN THE FOLLOWING WAYS:

Martin Day Publications
Secure On-Line Ordering at
www.MartinDayFitness.com

Snail Mail for ALL Correspondence and Orders:
Martin Day Publications
Suite 8, Noosa Boardroom
28 Eenie Creek Rd
Noosaville Queensland 4566, Australia

Call 24 hrs:

Within Australia
Tel: 1300 851 401
Fax: 07 5430 6677

International:
Phone: + 61 7 5430 6662
Fax: + 61 7 5430 6677

DEFEND YOURSELF!

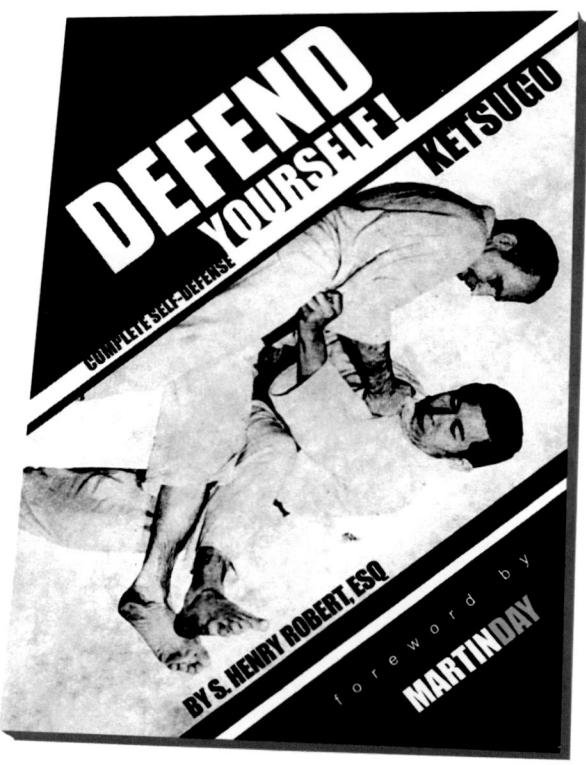

"Never Be Afraid Again—Learn How To Defend Yourself From Any Attack"

In the 8 chapters contained within this great book here's a snippet of what you'll learn:

• What Ketsugo is. Find out what this means and how it is going to help you survive any attack.

• How to condition the body, so that it is always ready to defend and counter-attack.

• Everything you need to know about keeping fit. You'll learn how to condition yourself and achieve awesome ability.

• What distraction is and how to use it in self defense. An important part of any martial art is knowing how to distract your opponent and then use devastating techniques to 'win'.

• How to use your attacker's weight against them. With this strategy, even a huge hulking brute can be defeated.

• All about the target area's and pressure points on a person's body. *You must be extremely careful here as you can render someone completely immobile or even kill them!*

• Details about the history of martial arts training systems including Karate, which has been in existence for thousands of years and has been proven to be a formidable way of protecting you, your family and your friends.
And there's loads more…

YOU CAN CONTACT US IN THE FOLLOWING WAYS:

Martin Day Publications
Secure On-Line Ordering at
www.MartinDayFitness.com

Snail Mail for ALL Correspondence and Orders:
Martin Day Publications
Suite 8, Noosa Boardroom
28 Eenie Creek Rd
Noosaville Queensland 4566, Australia

Call 24 hrs:

Within Australia
Tel: 1300 851 401
Fax: 07 5430 6677

International:
Phone: + 61 7 5430 6662
Fax: + 61 7 5430 6677

BASIC KATAS

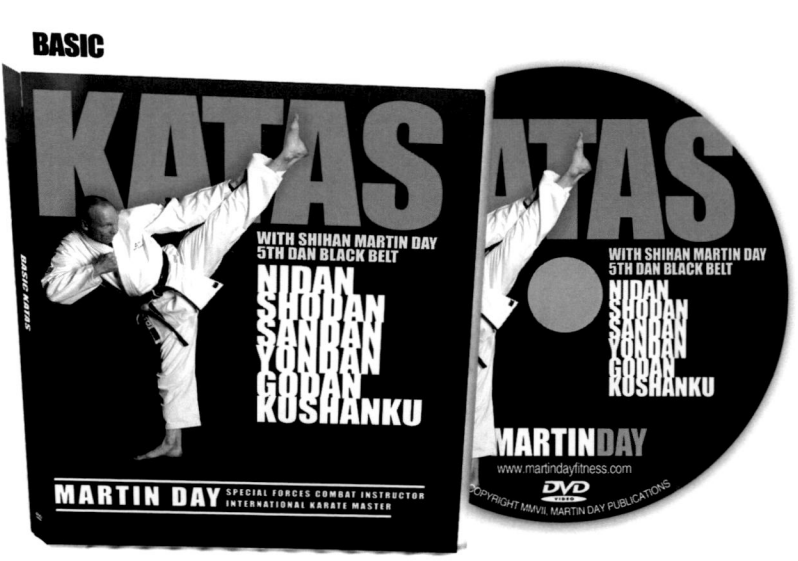

Katas are also known as Patterns or Forms.

Each of the six Martial Arts Katas are shown precisely and clearly and is then demonstrated close up with verbal explanations to allow the student to follow along. The most difficult aspects of each Kata are then demonstrated from a variety of angles.

International Karate Master Shihan Martin Day 5th Dan Black Belt, Founder and Chief Instructor of Combat Karate International demonstrates all of the Katas with an emphasis on technique, speed, power and flexibility that he is renowned for.

The DVD uses easy menus and chapters in order to select the Kata you wish to practice.

So if you are a beginner or seasoned martial artist or you have no experience in combat sports doesn't matter - this DVD will get you fit, co-ordinated and strong.

Katas that Martin Day has spent many years piecing together are:

Nidan, Shodan, Sandan, Yondan, Godan, Kushanku

YOU CAN CONTACT US IN THE FOLLOWING WAYS:

Martin Day Publications
Secure On-Line Ordering at
www.MartinDayFitness.com

Snail Mail for ALL Correspondence and Orders:
Martin Day Publications
Suite 8, Noosa Boardroom
28 Eenie Creek Rd
Noosaville Queensland 4566, Australia

Call 24 hrs:

Within Australia
Tel: 1300 851 401
Fax: 07 5430 6677

International:
Phone: + 61 7 5430 6662
Fax: + 61 7 5430 6677

ADVANCED BLACK BELT KATAS

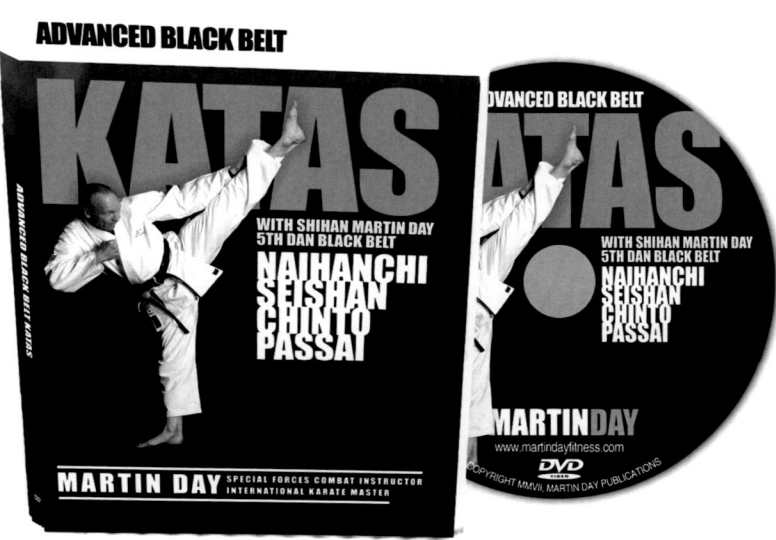

Naihanchi, Seishan, Chinto, Passai

This is another dynamic training DVD featuring Shihan Martin Day 5th Dan demonstrating advanced Black Belt Kata's.

He presents them in a way that is easy for intermediate and advanced students from any training system to follow and understand.

You will develop your martial arts training skills to an extremely HIGH level by watching and practicing along with this ground breaking DVD.

Each of the four Kata's is shown precisely and clearly and is then demonstrated close up and with verbal explanations.

So if it's a challenge that you are after and a different aspect on training then this DVD is for you.

YOU CAN CONTACT US IN THE FOLLOWING WAYS:

Martin Day Publications
Secure On-Line Ordering at
www.MartinDayFitness.com

Snail Mail for ALL Correspondence and Orders:

Martin Day Publications
Suite 8, Noosa Boardroom
28 Eenie Creek Rd
Noosaville Queensland 4566, Australia

Call 24 hrs:

Within Australia
Tel: 1300 851 401
Fax: 07 5430 6677

International:
Phone: + 61 7 5430 6662
Fax: + 61 7 5430 6677

SECRETS OF FIGHTING FIT EXPOSED

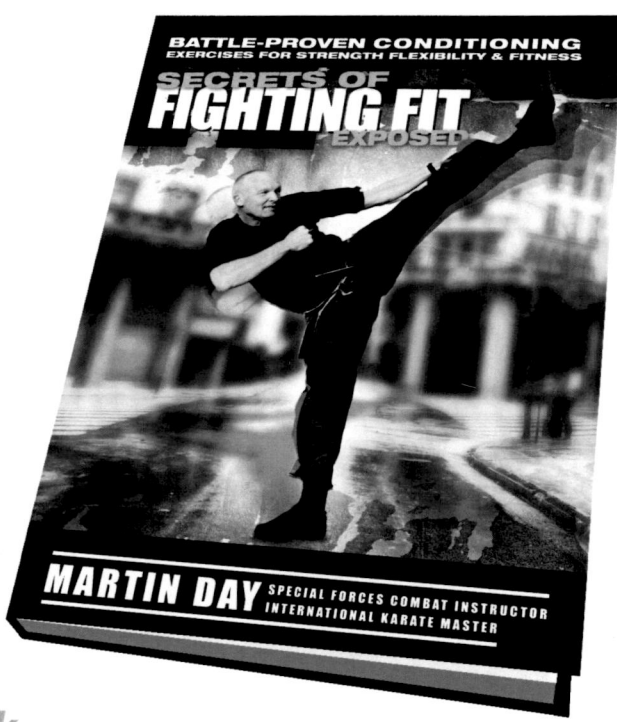

Sneak Peek......

SECRETS OF FIGHTING FIT EXPOSED BOOK

Battle- Proven Bodyweight Conditioning For Strength, Fitness & Flexibility…

This 160 page book is full of vital information gained over thirty years in Martin Day's service in the British Army and in his martial arts career. It includes the BATTLE GROUP series of unique exercises that guarantee success; so if it's losing weight, toning up, gaining functional strength and fitness then this book is for you!

My strength, fitness, power and flexibility have rocketed, enabling me to perform at my best both at work and in training. There is no doubt in my mind that my life has drastically changed for the better since as a direct result of implementing Martin Day's Fighting Fit training methods demonstrated in his book.

I urge all of you, no matter what your level of fitness, age and ability to give it a go!   *-* ***Simon Rowledge***

This best selling book has changed thousands of lives all over the world….

Martin Day Publications
Secure On-Line Ordering at
www.MartinDayFitness.com

Snail Mail for ALL Correspondence and Orders:
Martin Day Publications
Suite 8, Noosa Boardroom
28 Eenie Creek Rd
Noosaville Queensland 4566, Australia

Call 24 hrs:

Within Australia
Tel: 1300 851 401
Fax: 07 5430 6677

International:
Phone: + 61 7 5430 6662
Fax: + 61 7 5430 6677

MY NOTES

Just record anything that will assist in inspiring you to keep going.
My suggestion is to record training dates, times, exercises, sets, repetitions, your weight, your shape, your feelings (confidence) and your thoughts after completing your training sessions.

MY GOALS:

This is a great way for you to set your 'achievable' goals like I do so that you are successful in what you want to achieve now and in the future, go for this, don't delay and make sure you get it out of your head and written down here as soon as you can – don't hesitate, just do it.

You will be surprised at what you will achieve when your life goals are written down as it attracts universal 'positive forces' that are out there to help all of us........

Here they are:

Three months

....

....

....

....

Six months

....

....

....

....

Twelve months

....

....

....

....

Three years

....

....

....

....

Five years

....

....

....

....